Self-Assessment Colour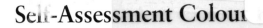

Reptiles and Amphibians

Fredric L. Frye
BSc, DVM, MSc, CBiol, FIBiol, FRSM
Davis, California

David L. Williams
MA, VetMB, CertVOphthal, MRCVS
Royal Veterinary College, London

Manson Publishing/The Veterinary Press

Copyright © 1995 Manson Publishing Ltd
ISBN 1–874545–32–4

A CIP catalogue record for this book is available from the British Library.

For full details of all Manson Publishing Ltd titles please write to Manson
Publishing Ltd, 73 Corringham Road, London NW11 7DL, UK.

Design and layout: Patrick Daly

Colour reproduction: Reed Reprographics, Ipswich, UK

Printed by: Grafos S.A., Barcelona, Spain

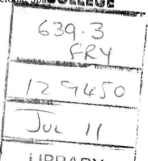
Cover illustration: A young adult male Jackson's Chameleon, *Chamaeleo Jacksoni*,
photographed by Dr F. L. Frye on the island of Maui, Hawaii, 1994.

Acknowledgements

The senior author wishes to express his heartfelt appreciation to Brucye Frye, who offered many constructive suggestions and edited the senior author's original manuscript as the cases were selected and the text was written.

Since its inception, this project has been a joy for both of us. We hope that those who peruse these pages and learn from these cases will gain the vital information that is necessary when diagnosing and treating the diverse reptilian and amphibian patients who often differ markedly from more conventional veterinary patients. It took 30 years to accumulate these cases. We urge our readers to make their cases available to others so that we may all increase our knowledge.

Michael Manson, managing director of Manson Publishing Limited, consistently showed great interest and enthusiasm in this project, and it was a genuine pleasure dealing with him and his entire editorial and production staff during the prepublication preparation of this book.

Several colleagues generously contributed images or specimens which illustrate this book. In alphabetical order, the following permitted the senior author to reproduce the following photographs and radiographs (identified by question numbers):

Dr. Alonso Aguirre: **191**.
Dr. Stephen L. Barten: **47** (page 36); **225** (pages 163 and 164); **258**.
Dr. Ralph F. Claxton: **130** (page 93).
Dr. Nathan W. Cohen: **76**.
Dr. James H. Corcoran: **48** (page 35, bottom left).
Dr. James Detterline: **46**; **194**.
Mr. Robin Houston: **2**.
Dr. Douglas R. Mader: **36**; **218**.
Dr. Scott McDonald: **83**; **123**; **131**.
Mr. and Mrs. J. E. Merrill: **166**.
Ms. Wendy Townsend: **116**.

The remaining images are the work of the authors.

Dedication

To Brucye and Jennie, Lorraine, Erik, Bice, Noah and Ian.

Introduction

This text was written with a retrospective view and deep appreciation of the history of comparative medicine and comparative pathology. Pioneers, such as the 18th century's John Hunter, and Rudolph Virchow, who died early this century, contributed mightily to our fund of knowledge; they were among the first physician-pathologists to realise the rationale of the commonsense approach of considering not only the solitary lesion but, more importantly, the intimate relationship of one condition, organ, or organ system to the well-being or disease of the entire organism. Of equal importance is that both of these giants of comparative medicine appreciated the value of teaching this approach to their contemporary health care professionals when explaining physiological interdependencies. This was revolutionary, even heretical, to many ears and was diametrically opposed to the dogma of that era. Hunter's and Virchow's philosophy was particularly enlightened when one considers that pathogenic bacteria, fungi, actinomycetes and viruses were only relatively recently discovered as the causes of infectious disease.

The patient must be seen as a whole, not merely the sum of his or her many disparate body parts. Balzac* observed that 'There are conflicts between diseases and physicians...of which physicians alone have any knowledge and whose reward in cases of success is never found in the paltry price of their labours nor, indeed, under the patient's roof but in the sweet gratification...bestowed upon true artists by the satisfaction they feel...in having acomplished a worthy work.' Those sentiments were as germane to veterinary surgeons as they were to human physicians and barber surgeons; and they are as appropriate today as they were well over a century-and-a-half ago (perhaps even more so) because today the healing arts have at their disposal so many more means for arriving at an accurate diagnosis and novel methods for treating diseases. Only after carefully assembling a history, keenly observing the patient's physical signs and conducting specialised investigations can a list of differential diagnoses be constructed; then, like kernels of grain, that list must be winnowed gradually until only one or, at most, a very few possibilities remain. From these, a prognosis is formulated; only then can a rational course of therapy or corrective surgery be established and carried out. Because of economic considerations, valuable clinical laboratory investigations may not always be executed, but most of these cases will not be diminished if enough required information has been gathered from the client and if the patient has been examined meticulously. By completing each task conscientiously and consistently, the probability of success is enhanced. In this self-assessment guide we have provided sufficient explicit information from which to formulate differential diagnoses, decide upon treatment plans and arrive at prognoses. The clues to the solution of clinical puzzles are often subtle. When examining radiographs and electrocardiograms, you may find surprises lurking, ready to snag the unwary. In some instances, the diagnosis is obvious, but the prognosis or treatment might not be so clear. This approach was taken because in real life situations the diagnosis and treatment of patients are not always trouble-free or easily achieved. We have systematically decreased the number of provisional diagnoses by proposing various

*Balzac, Honoré de. (1840). *Pierrette*. Ives, GB transl. (1897), Geo Barrie & Sons, Philadelphia, 215-216.

reasonable explanations, when necessary. Several things must be understood: not all clients tell the whole truth; some may not actually lie about their animals, but also they may not always volunteer details that might be vitally important to the final diagnosis and outcome of their particular case; others may, for their own reasons, conceal facts that might be germane. As mentioned before, economics often plays a major role in how an animal responds to treatment – or whether it is even examined and treated professionally – particularly if the definitive diagnosis relies upon expensive tests or procedures. We have selected cases which are instructive and probably would/could be seen in clinical practice. The majority are common everyday cases; a few are exotic and may have been observed only once. For those readers who have never observed even a single example of one of the common everyday cases, the purchase of this text is justified; the rarer cases are included to whet the intellectual appetites of the more experienced of our readers. Perhaps, just perhaps, a similar puzzling case will arrive on your doorstep one day; having experienced the question and answer vicariously in the pages of this guide may make your case all the more memorable! The popularity of certain reptiles as pets or study animals is reflected in the selection of cases for this book; it is for this reason that so many iguanas are included as representatives of reptilian disease. Some people who possess large, showy and expressive lizards are often willing and able to incur the considerable expense of having their pets properly diagnosed and treated; others who own another species of herbivorous lizard perceived as being of less value may elect not to have it examined and evaluated. However, we are confident that information regarding the physiological responses to disease in iguanas is sufficiently similar to disease processes in other herbivorous lizards. Bacterial infections, parasitism and many metabolic disorders in North American chelonians closely mimic the same conditions observed in European, African or Asian turtles, terrapins and tortoises and *vice versa*. We have included more than a single case of some particular conditions (but each has differed somewhat) because we believe that repeating the discussion of these common, but significant, conditions is important due to their ramifications; in these instances we have endeavoured to include special features that will maintain your interest. We wish to enunciate one caveat: 'normal' values are only rarely cited in this guide. Unlike humans and domestic animals, from which thousands of data have been collected and collated, reptiles and especially captive reptiles (1) may or may not be normal (or even healthy) when their body fluids are sampled, and (2) the very nature of captivity and the stress incurred during restraint in order to obtain the samples introduce variables that are reflected in the laboratory results. We recognise these shortcomings and urge the reader to consider these undeniable facts when judging whether a laboratory finding is meaningful or out of 'normal' range. (We used only the most current 'accurate' values available, but advise you to keep your sceptic's salt-shaker at the ready!)

Fredric L Frye
David L Williams
January 1995

English and Latin names

English	Latin
African bullfrog	*Pyxicephalus adspersus*
African clawed frog	*Xenopus laevis*
African leopard tortoise	*Geochelone pardalis*
Agama lizard	*Agama* sp.
American alligator	*Alligator mississippiensis*
American bullfrog	*Rana catesbiana*
Anaconda snake	*Eunectes marinus*
Argentine horned frog	*Ceratophrys oranata*
Asian box turtle	*Cuora amboinensis*
Asian red-tailed rat snake	*Gonysoma oxycephala*
Asian water dragon lizard	*Physignathus concincinus*
Australian bearded dragon lizard	*Pogona vitticeps*
Australian taipan	*Oxyuranus scutellatus*
Axolotl	*Ambystoma* sp.
Blanding's turtle	*Clemmys blandingi*
Blood python	*Python curtus*
Boa constrictor	*Boa constrictor constrictor*
Box turtle	*Terrapene carolina*
Burmese python	*Python molurus bivittatus*
California king snake	*Lampropeltis getulus californiae*
Caribbean rhinoceros iguana	*Cyclura nubila lewisii*
Carolina anole lizard	*Anolis carolinensis*
Children's python	*Liasis childreni*
Chilean tortoise	*Geochelone chilensis*
Chuckwalla lizard	*Sauromalus obesus*
Collared lizard	*Crotaphytus collaris*
Common iguana	*Iguana iguana*
Copperhead snake	*Agkistrodon contortrix*
Corn snake	*Elaphe guttata*
Desert tortoise	*Xerobates agassizzi*
Diamondback terrapin	*Malaclemys terrapin*
East African chameleon	*Chamaeleo dilepsis*
East African Fischer's chameleon	*Chamaeleo fischeri*
East African pancake tortoise	*Malacochersus tornieri*
Emerald tree boa	*Corralus caninus*
European green lizard	*Lacerta viridis*
Fence lizard	*Sceloporous occidentalis*
Gaboon viper	*Bitis gabonica*
Galapagos tortoise	*Geochelone elephantopus*
Garter snake	*Thamnophis sirtalis*
Giant blue-tongued skink	*Tiliqua gigas*
Gila monster lizard	*Heloderma suspectum*
Gopher snake	*Pituophis melanoleucus catenifer*
Gopher tortoise	*Gopherus polyphemus*
Green sea turtle	*Chelonia mydas*
Ground iguana	*Cyclura cornuta*
Hermann's tortoise	*Testudo hermanni*
Hog-nosed snake	*Heterodan platyrhinos*
Indigo snake	*Drymarchon corais*

Jackson's chameleon	*Chamaeleo jacksoni*
Javanese file snake	*Acrochordus javanicus*
King snake	*Lampropeltis getulus*
Leopard gecko	*Eublepharis macularius*
Malagasy tree boa	*Sanzinia madagascariensis*
	Boa mandrita
Mangrove monitor lizard	*Varanus indicus*
Map turtle	*Graptemys* sp.
Mata mata turtle	*Chelys fimbriatus*
Mexican dwarf python	*Loxocemus bicolor*
Nile monitor lizard	*Varanus niloticus*
North American banded king snake	*Lampropeltis alterna*
Pacific pond turtle	*Clemmys marmorata*
Rat snake	*Elaphe* sp.
Rattlesnake	*Crotalus atrox*
Red tegu lizard	*Tupinambis rufescens*
Red-eared slider turtle	*Trachemys scripta elegans*
Red-eyed frog	*Agalychnis callidryas*
Red-legged tortoise	*Geochelone carbonaria*
Reeve's turtle	*Chinemys reevesi*
Reticulated python	*Python reticulatus*
Rhinoceros iguana	*Cyclura nubila*
Rhinoceros viper	*Bitis nasicornis*
Rosy boa	*Lichanura trivirgata*
Royal python	*Python regius*
Russell's viper	*Vipera russelli*
Savannah monitor lizard	*Varanus exanthematicus*
Snapping turtle	*Chelydra serpentina*
Soft-shelled turtle	*Apalone* sp.
Solomon Island skink	*Corucia zebrata*
Spectacled caiman	*Caiman sclerops*
Spiny-tailed iguana	*Ctenosaurus* sp.
Tegu lizard	*Tupinambis teguixin*
Texas tortoise	*Xerobates berlandieri*
Timor monitor lizard	*Varanus timorensis*
Tokay gecko	*Gekko gekko*
Tree boa	*Corallus* sp.
Tree frog	*Pseudachris (hyla) regilla*
Vine snake	*Oxybelis aeneus*
Water monitor lizard	*Varanus salvator*
Water snake	*Nerodia (natrix) cyclopion*
Western painted turtle	*Chrysemys picta belli*
Western terrestrial garter snake	*Thamnophis sirtalis terrestris*
Western toad	*Bufo boreas halophilus*

1 i. What are the two oph-thalmic conditions affecting the eye of this elderly tortoise?
ii. How would you manage this case?

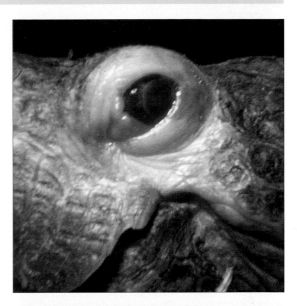

2 All of the snakes in a large collection are found to be infested with this small dark brown-to-black invertebrate that crawls about on the surface of the snakes' skin.
i. What is this creature?
ii. What is its significance?
iii. How would you treat this infestation?

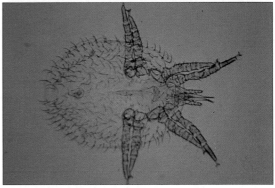

3 During mask induction of anaesthesia many reptiles engage in prolonged breath-holding and, under varying environmental conditions, they can survive even very low oxygen saturation in their inspired air.
i. Describe the metabolic processes by which reptiles are able to achieve these 'oxygen debts'.
ii. What is the significance of these processes?

1 i. *Arcus senilis* and chronic hypertrophy of the *membrana nictitans*.

ii. *Arcus senilis* is caused by deposition of cholesterol and other lipids or lipoids within the interstices of the corneal stroma and is thought to be age-related; thus, this lesion does not call for aggressive treatment. Chronic hypertrophy of the nictitating membrane is treated by thorough lavage of the conjunctival space, followed by instillation of a corticosteroid-containing antibiotic ophthalmic ointment two to three times daily.

2 i. A snake mite.

ii. These arthropod parasites must take a blood meal in order to reproduce. If sufficient numbers are present they can cause anaemia and substantial disturbance, and also peri-spectacular lesions, to the snakes upon which they feed.

iii. Soaking the affected snakes in slightly tepid water for 30 minutes daily will remove the majority of these mites. Spray a small quantity of a flea and tick spray that is formulated for kittens and puppies onto a clean cloth, and then let the snakes crawl through the moistened area, thus distributing a small amount onto their integument. The cages and all cage furniture must also be thoroughly cleaned and treated with an appropriate miticide so that the snakes do not become reinfested with mites.

3 i. Some reptiles are capable of sustaining significantly low oxygen levels by employing anaerobic respiration by the use of lactic acid as an energy source in their physiological tissue respiration. Others can exchange their respiratory gases through non-pulmonary mechanisms, such as cloacal respiration in aquatic environments.

ii. Many reptiles will engage in breath-holding if anaesthesia is initiated by mask induction. One method for overcoming this behaviour is to begin the induction with oxygen and nitrous oxide in equal amounts for the first few minutes before introducing a volatile gas such as isoflurane.

4 This lateral view radiograph is of a wild-caught ground iguana.
i. What is your diagnosis?
ii. How would you treat this condition?

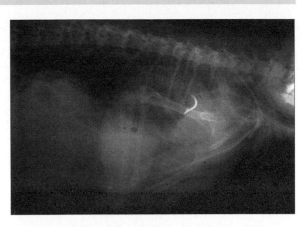

5 What ophthalmic condition is depicted in this boa's eye?

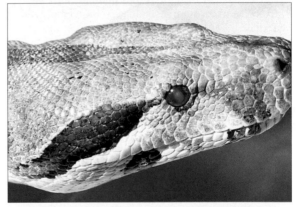

6 This box turtle is reluctant to walk. There is no history or evidence of trauma.
i. What is your tentative diagnosis?
ii. What test(s) would you perform to confirm your diagnosis?
iii. How would you treat this turtle?

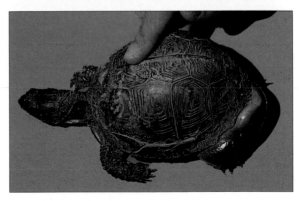

4 i. A foreign body (fish hook) is present within the thoracic portion of the coelomic cavity.

ii. Endoscopic oesophagoscopy did not reveal this object. During a thoracotomy, an abscess containing much pus and the fish hook was found in the subvertebral musculature. The broken fish hook had passed through the dorsal wall of the stomach and had embedded itself in the muscle. A block of muscle together with the abscess was excised; the thoracic cavity was lavaged thoroughly; a drain was installed; the thoracic wall was closed; and the lungs were inflated. The thoracic drain tube was removed on the sixth postoperative day. Broad-spectrum bacteriocidal antibiotics were administered for two weeks.

The iguana made an uneventful recovery and lived for several years after the thoracotomy. The presence of the fish hook is strong presumptive evidence that the iguana was wild-caught and had acquired the fish hook when he found and consumed a dead fish as carrion.

5 Early lenticular cataract.

6 i. Massive abscessation of soft tissues surrounding the left hindlimb.

ii. Cytological examination, Gram staining, and microbiological culture and sensitivity testing of exudate aspirated from the mass.

iii. Incision, drainage and thorough lavage of the abscess; parenteral bacteriocidal antibiobic therapy; and protection of the patient from flies while the open incision heals.

7 This large parasitic ovum was found in the faeces of an Anaconda snake.
i. What is your diagnosis?
ii. How would you treat the snake for this parasite?

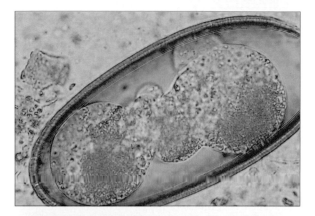

8 The coelomic cavity of an adult male iguana.
i. What is your diagnosis?
ii. What can cause this condition?

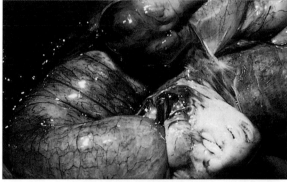

9 i. Identify the white structure on the rostrum of this hatchling tortoise.
ii. What is the function of this structure?

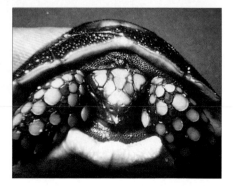

10 Some reptile species, such as garter snakes, feed exclusively or predominately upon fish. Under wild, natural conditions this poses no difficulty because the fish are usually alive when caught and eaten. However, when improperly-stored frozen and thawed fat-laden fish are fed to captive animals, what dietary deficiencies are likely consequences?

7 i. Hookworm ovum.
ii. Effective treatment would be ivermectin (200mcg/kg i/m or orally, repeated in two weeks); or pyrantel pamoate (5mg/kg, repeated in two weeks); or levamisol HCl (5 mg/kg, repeated in two weeks); or febendazole (50–100mg/kg, repeated in two weeks).

8 i. An intussusception.
ii. Intussusceptions are induced by irritation and inflammation of bowel segments, gastrointestinal parasitism, and foreign bodies.

9 i. A caruncle, or 'egg-tooth.'
ii. This sharp structure is used to slit or 'pip' the eggshell, and enables the hatchling to escape the confines of the eggshell. The caruncle drops off a day or two after the tortoise hatches.

10 Hypovitaminosis B_1 (thiamine) and hypovitaminosis E. Thiamine deficiency is induced as a result of the action of the lytic enzyme, thiaminase, often present in the flesh of improperly stored fish, shellfish and some plants.The photomicrograph (**below**) is of the brain from an induced thiaminase vitamin B_1 deficiency caused by feeding improperly stored fish. Note the extensive demyelination seen as numerous clear spaces and loss of dense blue staining. (Luxol fast blue stain, x67 original magnification).

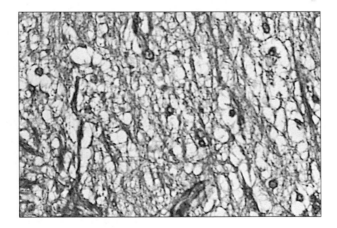

11 A 1.4kg young adult male iguana that had previously been thriving presented with anorexia which had begun approximately two weeks before its owners found their pet upside-down on the bottom of its cage, apparently dead. However, when they prodded it, the iguana responded by moving its limbs feebly. Clinical examination manifested a severely depressed iguana whose integument and oral mucous membranes were icteric; its eyes were deeply sunken. No grossly visible lesions or palpable swellings or masses were present. Ultrasonic Doppler blood-flow studies detected bilateral loud atrioventricular and aortic valvular murmurs. The diet was composed primarily of collard, mustard, turnip and dandelion greens with occasional soft fresh fruit. The pre-treatment specimen of blood was very dark red and its flow into the syringe was substantially slower than normal; it clotted almost immediately. The results of the haematology and clinical biochemical tests are listed below:

Test	Value
Haematocrit (%)	62
WBC (/mm³)	13,000
Heterophils (%)	83
Lymphocytes (%)	13
Monocytes (%)	2
Azurophils (%)	2
Thrombocytes	adequate
Glucose (mg/dl)	591
SGPT (ALT) (iu/l)	30
SGOT (AST) (iu/l)	114
Creatinine phosphokinase (CPK)	1731
LDH (iu/l)	1110
Alkaline phosphatase (iu/l)	0
Cholesterol (mg/dl)	357
Calcium (mg/dl)	14.7
Phosphorus (mg/dl)	18.9
Total protein (mg/dl)	9.3
Albumin (mg/dl)	2.4
Globulin (mg/dl)	6.9
A/G ratio	0.4
Sodium (mEq/l)	123
Potassium (mEq/l)	15.3
Uric acid (mg/dl)	69.6
BUN (mg/dl)	6.0
Creatinine	0.6

i. Based upon the brief clinical narrative and the laboratory results, what would be your initial treatment of this iguana?
ii. How do you interpret the pathogenesis of the elevated CPK enzyme value and, in light of the potassium and sodium levels, what special precautions would you take with this patient?
iii. How do you interpret the BUN, creatinine, uric acid, calcium and phosphorus levels in this iguana? How might these determinations alter your treatment?
iv. Would you expect this iguana to be capable of mounting an adequate immunogenic response to its underlying condition? If affirmative, why? If negative, why?

11 i. The presence of deeply sunken eyes, and the results of the haematology and clinical biochemistry tests that indicated markedly elevated haematocrit, total protein, potassium, phosphorus, and uric acid levels, demand immediate expansion of the plasma volume to re-establish renal perfusion and to lessen the stress on the cardiovascular and pulmonary systems. Massive hyperkalaemia would usually be inconsistent with life; indeed, this iguana was near death when it was first presented for examination and evaluation.

ii. The elevated CPK enzyme level was probably directly related to the greatly increased myocardial exertion induced by the increase in blood viscosity. The haematocrit was approximately 50% greater than is normal, and in order for the heart to pump this viscous fluid, it was forced to work much harder. It is likely that pulmonary function was probably impaired; therefore, some degree of hypoxaemia was present when the blood was drawn and this also may have contributed to the elevated CPK. Because of the markedly elevated plasma potassium and the low plasma sodium, physiologic saline was infused (35ml i/v and 65ml intracoelomically) rather than Ringer's solution. It was imperative that the fluid did not contain potassium ions. Within less than five minutes following infusion, the iguana became more animated. One hour after the fluid was administered, the haematocrit had decreased to 42%. By the next morning, it had decreased to 34% and the heart and blood flow murmurs were no longer detected with the Doppler instrument, and the iguana was actively thrashing his tail at the personnel trying to treat him!

iii. The normal BUN and creatinine levels concomitant with the extremely elevated uric acid level demonstrate clearly that only uric acid is a meaningful determinant of renal function in terrestrial reptiles. Although the plasma calcium was normal, the plasma phosphorus was approximately three times higher than normal. This hyperphosphataemia is a reflection of renal retention of phosphorus. Had the loss of kidney function been more severe or more chronic, it is likely that the plasma calcium level would have been substantially lower, because as hyperphosphataemia stimulates the parathyroid glands to secrete parathormone (PTH), bone stores of calcium are mobilised, eventually resulting in renal-associated osteomalacia (metabolic bone disease, fibrous osteodystrophy, 'rubber jaw', etc). Due to the hyperphosphataemia, the iguana was placed on a regimen of saline diuresis maintained at 45ml/kg daily in two divided doses, plus as much oral fluid as it would accept without developing oedema and/or ascites. Enzymatic diuresis was not employed because the iguana tolerated the saline diuresis well and voided abundant urates and fluid urine.

iv. Yes. Evidence of adequate cell-mediated and humeral antibody-mediated immune responses were reflected by the marked heterophilia and globulin values. A course of parenteral enrofloxacin was initiated on the first day of hospitalisation, and was later changed to oral doses of enrofloxacin when the iguana was released for home treatment. The iguana made an uneventful recovery. The final diagnosis was subacute bacterial nephritis. The causes for the hyperglycaemia and hypercholesterolaemia were not determined conclusively.

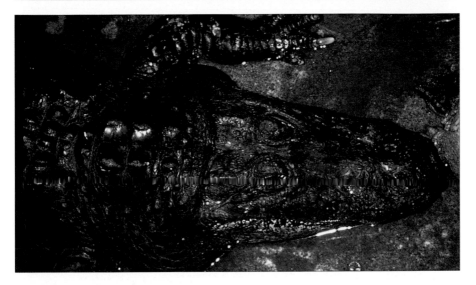

12 This adult female American alligator has multiple pink-to-grey moist lesions on the skin of its head, neck and limbs.
i. What are your differential diagnoses?
ii. What tests would you perform to help confirm your diagnosis?
iii. How would you treat this condition?

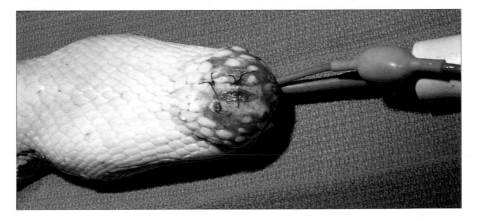

13 A mature female Burmese python develops a progressively enlarging mass that originated on her mandible. Within a few weeks, the gingiva rolled outward because the underlying mandibular bone became so distorted.
i. What is your diagnosis?
ii. How would you treat this snake?
iii. What is the prognosis?

12 i. (1) Bacterial dermatitis, (2) mycotic dermatitis and (3) acute trauma.

ii. Specimens for microbiological culture and sensitivity testing should be obtained, and a small piece of a typical lesion should be biopsied for histopathological examination. In this instance, mycology yielded *Penicillium* sp. in pure culture (**right**).

iii. Treat by initially cleansing the integument

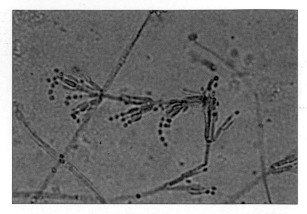

with dilute povidone iodine solution. Then, topically apply ketoconazole cream twice daily, and administer oral ketoconazole daily at a dosage of 10–30mg/kg (by inserting ketoconazole tablets in small food items) for at least two weeks. The alligator should be kept dry during this treatment except for brief periods when it can eat and drink.

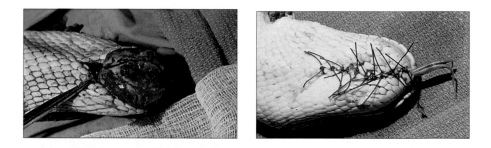

13 i. Neoplasia. The histopathological diagnosis in this case was fibrosarcoma.

ii. If feasible, the mass should be removed *in toto*. If this cannot be achieved, as much of the mass as possible should be removed (**see above**) and the balance, as well as the bed from which it arises, should be subjected to at least three freeze-thaw cycles of cryosurgery.

iii. The prognosis is guarded. The mass was excised and the subjacent tissue was treated with cryosurgery, as described above. The python lived for 23 months before she died with widely disseminated metastatic tumours. This longevity was unexpected and characterises the often bizarre behaviour of some reptilian neoplasms that would be rapidly fatal if they occurred in a mammal.

14 i. Describe the ophthalmic condition affecting the left eye of this rat snake.
ii. What caused this condition?
iii. How would you treat this snake?

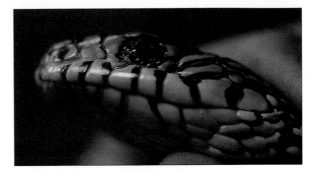

15 This Blanding's turtle displays a head tilt and circles to its left.
i. What is your interpretation of the clinical signs exhibited by this turtle?
ii. What is the likely cause?
iii. How would you treat this turtle?

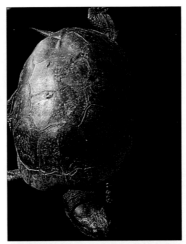

16 The adult newt shown at the upper left had an acute onset of coelomic distention. When placed into a few centimetres of water, the newt immediately floated to the surface and could not dive. There was no history or evidence of trauma. Treatment initiated by the veterinarian brought immediate relief and was continued at home by the owner. Within two weeks the newt recovered completely.
i. What is your diagnosis?
ii. What was the treatment?

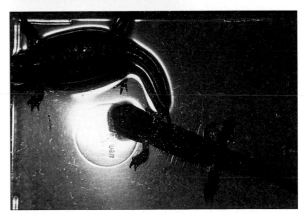

14 i. Avulsion of the tertiary spectacle and underlying cornea, with exposure of the contents of the globe.
ii. An injudicious attempt to remove a retained spectacle without prior moisturisation of the retained spectacle.
iii. The eye is irreparably damaged and should be enucleated.

15 i. Vestibular syndrome.
ii. Abscess-inducing, extracranial pressure on the caudolateral region of the skull and cranial cervical soft tissues.
iii. Evacuate and drain the inflammatory lesion under general anaesthesia; obtain a specimen of the exudate for microbiological culture and sensitivity testing; flush the abscess cavity with 0.75% chlorhexidine solution; and commence a course of parenteral bacteriocidal antibiotic therapy.

16 i. Acute pulmonary emphysema from a spontaneously ruptured pulmonary bulla.
ii. Escaped air was aspirated from within the coelomic cavity with a very fine hypodermic needle and disposable syringe once or twice daily. Within a few days less and less air was escaping, and within two weeks the newt was normal again. The aetiology of the emphysema is unclear. Once the extrapulmonary air had been removed, the leaks in the pulmonary tissue closed and the lungs healed.

17 i. What ophthalmic condition is depicted in this turtle?
ii. What is the treatment?

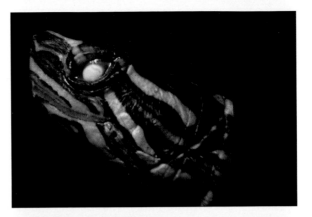

18 This male snake is unable to retract one of his hemipenes into the post-cloacal sheath on one side of his tail.
i. What is your diagnosis?
ii. What might be some of the potential aetiologies for this disorder?
iii. How should this condition be managed?

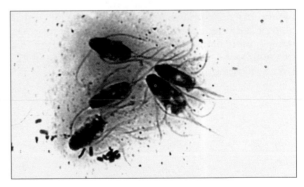

19 The photomicrograph is of a wet mount of several organisms found in the turbid coelomic fluid aspirated from a severely depressed Pacific pond turtle. What is your diagnosis?

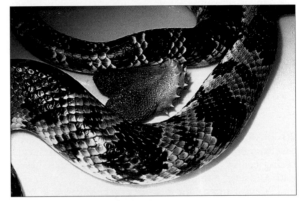

20 An adult female royal python has refused to feed voluntarily for several months beginning in early September.
i. How do you interpret this behaviour?
ii. What measures would you take to help remedy this prolonged anorexia?

17–20: Answers

17 i. Coagulative keratopathy.
ii. Topical instillation of an ophthalmic ointment containing a proteolytic enzyme. These lesions usually clear within a week of conservative topical therapy.

18 i. Prolapse of a hemipenis.
ii. One or both hemipenes may prolapse as a result of irritation or inflammation of the organ(s) or their sheath tissues, incarceration of the phallus by a foreign body such as a hair, the loss of neural control of the retractor penis muscle(s), or trauma to one or both retractor penis muscles.
iii. If possible, the prolapsed organ(s) should be cleansed and replaced back into its sheath(s). However, the prolapsed organ is often severely engorged and indurated; the topical application of glycerine or concentrated sucrose solution (not dry granules) may reduce the swelling sufficiently to permit a well lubricated hemipenis to be replaced. A purse-string suture is inserted in the pericloacal vent rim just tightly enough to prevent reprolapse but sufficiently loose to permit passage of urinary wastes and small stool boluses. The suture is usually kept in place for one week. If the prolapsed organ exhibits evidence of paralysis, infection, maceration or severe trauma, or if it cannot be replaced, amputation is necessary. If only one hemipenis is lost, the animal can still serve as a breeder.

19 Hexamitosis. The flagella-bearing organisms are *Hexamita* spp.

20 i. Although not all royal pythons exhibit this behaviour, many refuse to feed for several months, particularly during the autumn in northern latitudes (corresponds to spring below the equator, which is the normal breeding time in the royal python's native African habitat).
ii. The most important measures to be taken are: make certain that the captive habitat is clean; provide the necessary fresh water container and 'hide box' into which the python can seek refuge; keep the environment satisfactorily warm and moderately humid; and offer appropriate rodent prey. In their native habitat, royal pythons prey upon agouti-coloured jerds; thus, they may refuse to feed upon white mice and rats. Metronidazole at a non-therapeutic oral dosage of 12.5mg/kg can be given to stimulate the flagging appetite.

21 This female gopher snake has displayed anorexia for approximately four weeks, and there are noticeable swellings in the caudal coelomic cavity.
i. What is your diagnosis?
ii. What is your treatment for this condition?

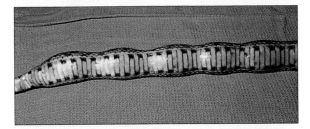

22 This soft-shelled turtle has been fed a diet of nothing but chopped raw beef heart and lamb kidney for over six months. It is now weak and depressed.
i. What is your diagnosis?
ii. How would you treat this condition?
iii. What advice would you give to the owner to help prevent this disorder from recurring?

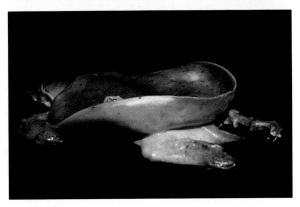

23 A knowledge of the gross and regional anatomy of reptiles is important because anaesthetic, surgical and clinical medical methods rely upon understanding where certain organs are located. Reptiles generally have paired lungs. Which reptiles (with few exceptions) have only a solitary lung?

24 When you are handling amphibians, why is it important always to wear wet latex gloves?

25 With respect to sex determination, why is the incubation temperature of all crocodilian, many chelonian, and some lizard eggs important?

26 Why is the parasiticide ivermectin not recommended for use in tortoises and turtles?

21 i. Gravidity. The snake is carrying maturing shelled eggs.
ii. Providing a suitable nesting place in which the snake can deposit her eggs is often all that is required. If a snake fails to deposit her eggs after an appropriate length of time, it may be necessary to administer either oxytocin (2 units/kg i/m) or arginine-, aminosuberic arginine-, or lysine-vasotocin (0.1–1.0mcg/kg i/m). A modest dose of parenteral calcium gluconate or calcium borogluconate (1.0–2.5mg/kg) may be administered one to two hours before the hormone is administered to promote its effects. If, for some reason, the snake fails to respond to conservative treatment, the eggs may have to be removed surgically via a salpingotomy.

22 i. Metabolic bone disease due to secondary nutritional hyperparathyroidism, induced by being fed a diet overly rich in phosphorus and grossly deficient in available calcium.
ii. Parenteral calcium gluconate or lactate (1.0–2.5mg/kg daily) and **oral** vitamin D_3 (1–4 iu/kg daily).
iii. Change the diet to a more natural ration consisting of small live fish, freshly excavated earthworms, and/or a commercial nutritionally balanced turtle or trout chow.

23 Most snakes possess only one functional lung. Often, the other lung is lacking altogether, or represented as only a non-respiratory remnant. Chelonians, lizards, crocodilians and the tuatara have paired lungs.

24 To prevent trauma to the amphibians' delicate and mucoid integument. Even the fine ridges and whorls comprising human fingerprints can damage the sensitive skin covering many aquatic and semi-aquatic amphibians. Once this natural barrier is breached, pathogens are afforded an opportunity to cause infections.

25 The sex determination of all crocodilians, many chelonians and some lizards is epigenetic rather than genetic: it is the temperature at which the developing embryos within fertilised eggs are incubated that determines the eventual sex of the neonate. Therefore, heterogametic sex determination does not occur in these reptiles.

26 Although ivermectin is highly effective in most reptiles, it has often proved to be lethally toxic to chelonians.

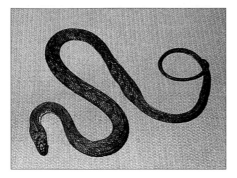

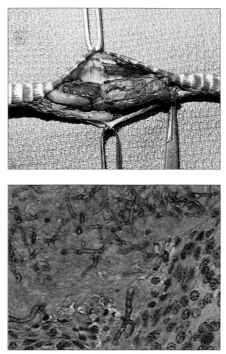

27 An adult female water snake develops a firm, caudal, intra-coelomic swelling in the region of its kidneys (**top, left**). Exploratory coeliotomy reveals both kidneys to be pale pink, massively swollen, and granular in appearance (**top, right**). Stained impression smears of the renal tissue discloses the presence of filamentous structures containing internal compartments separated by transverse walls (**right**). What is your diagnosis?

28 You have a profoundly anaemic iguana patient and do not have access to another iguana that could serve as a blood donor.
i. Would the blood obtained from a large frog or pigeon be a rational substitute?
ii. If so, for how long would you anticipate the heterologous erythrocytes to survive in the iguana?
iii. If, in your opinion, giving a heterologous transfusion would not be appropriate, why not?
iv. What alternative measures could you take to treat this anaemic iguana?

29 Amphibians and reptiles possess a vascular system that differs markedly from that of a mammalian vascular system.
i. What is the single greatest difference found in the vascular path taken in these so-called 'lower' vertebrates?
ii. Why is this difference of clinical importance when treating amphibians and reptiles?

30 Many diurnal reptiles bask in sunlight in order to increase their deep-core body temperature. During this behaviour, vitamin D_3 is synthesised by endogenous means. Which organs/tissues are essential to the process of vitamin D_3 synthesis?

27 Bilateral renal mycetoma. The organism is *Aspergillus* sp.

28 i. No.
ii. Investigations using radioactive Cr^{51}-tagged avian erythrocytes have shown that heterologous transfusions of one bird's blood into a different species of bird result in survival for only a few hours. Thus, avian RBCs are expected to survive for only a similarly brief time in an iguana.
iii. No. Heterologous erythrocytes would be removed quickly from the vascular pool by the reticulo-endothelial system and impose a further physiological stress on an already labile patient.
iv. Oxygenate the patient.

29 i. Amphibians and reptiles possess renal portal veins which direct a portion of the venous blood draining the caudal portion of the body through the renal circulation before it enters the hepatic circulation.
ii. Because of the renal portal venous drainage, it is (theoretically) possible when injecting nephrotoxic drugs into the hind quarters or caudal portions of an amphibian or reptile to deliver a bolus of concentrated drug to the kidneys. Although in practice this is probably a rare occurrence, it is always wise to inject potentially nephrotoxic agents into the cranial half of the body.

30 In reptiles, the dynamic synthesis of vitamin D_3 involves all of the following organs and tissues, some directly, others via feedback loops: skin, liver, kidney, parathyroid gland, thyroid interfollicular 'C' cells, and bone. This process is particularly important in diurnal reptiles that display basking in their behavioural repertoire. Nocturnally active, fossorial (burrowing) and crepuscular (active only at dusk or during times of subdued light) species rely upon preformed vitamin D contained in their diet rather than synthesising their own endogenously. Because of these differences, it may be necessary to supplement the diet of some reptiles with preformed vitamin D_3 if they are not exposed regularly to a source of suitable quality ultraviolet light.

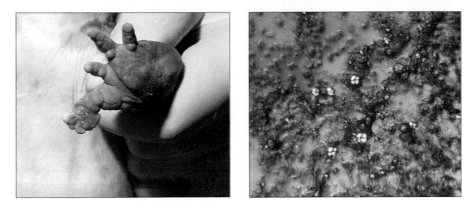

31 The swollen toe of an African bullfrog (**above, left**). The photomicrograph (**above, right**) is of a wet preparation made from the material contained within the swelling.
i. What is your diagnosis?
ii. How would you treat this condition?

32 You make a venepuncture into the tail base of a chameleon and withdraw clear, straw-coloured fluid. Explain what has happened.

33 Rapidly growing, juvenile lizards often develop metabolic bone disease as a result of which of the following imbalances or deficiencies?
i. Vitamin A deficiency and vitamin D excess.
ii. Vitamin C excess and vitamin E deficiency.
iii. Vitamin B_1 deficiency and vitamin D excess.
iv. Vitamin D deficiency with phosphorus deficiency.
v. Vitamin D deficiency with calcium deficiency.

34 i. Identify the ophthalmic disorder evident in this immature tree boa.
ii. How would you treat this condition?

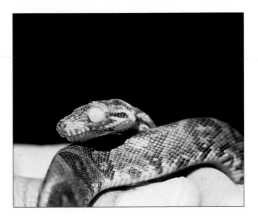

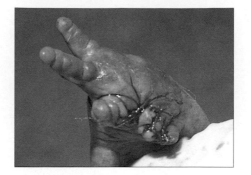

31 i. Articular and periarticular gout.

ii. Because this was a solitary lesion confined to a single digit, the entire toe was amputated at its palmar attachment. The picture (**above**) shows the postoperative appearance of the surgical site. The entire digit was excised, leaving two curvilinear flaps that were apposed and sutured over the surgical defect.

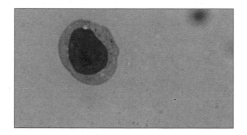

32 The lymph 'heart' or a major lymphatic vessel has been entered. These vascular-like structures are characteristic of the caudal anatomy of many reptiles. When this occurs, withdraw the needle, discard the clear lymph, and try to obtain blood from another site. **Above** is a photomicrograph of a lymphocyte in a specimen of lymph. Note the pale grey-blue cytoplasm and large central nucleus.

33 v. Vitamin D deficiency with calcium deficiency.

34 i. Sub-spectacular empyema.

ii. Anaesthetise the boa; clean the tertiary spectacle and the surrounding integument; make a small incision through the distended spectacle; introduce a sterile needle into the interspectacular-corneal space; flush the cavity with 0.75% chlorhexidine solution until the space has been cleared of all exudate; then instill a bacteriocidal antibiotic solution or ointment daily until healed or until the snake moults and loses the diseased spectacle. If this does not fully ameliorate the condition a 30° wedge resection of the ventral spectacle will allow a more prolonged drainage of the purulent material.

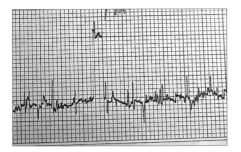

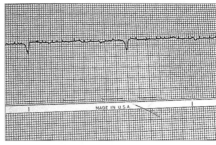

35 This ornamental plant (right) was consumed by an adult desert tortoise. An ECG (top, left) was obtained approximately 45 minutes after the tortoise had ingested a few leaves of this plant. A further ECG (top, right) was obtained 30 minutes after the tortoise was treated.
i. Identify this plant.
ii. What are the major abnormalities revealed by the ECG?
iii. What is a rational treatment for the condition affecting the tortoise?

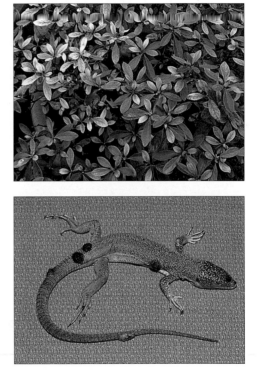

36 This European green lizard has multiple, raised, inky-dark integumentary lesions.
i. What is your diagnosis?
ii. Are these lesions infectious?
iii. What is the treatment for this condition?

37 When injecting an aminoglycoside antibiotic, or other nephrotoxic agents, into reptiles, the preferred site is in the cranial half of the body because of peculiarities in which of the following reptilian vascular systems?
i. Splanchnic venous system.
ii. Renal portal system.
iii. Hepatic portal system.
iv. Coronary artery system.

35 i. An azalea. Like other members of the Ericaceae family, azaleas contain the cardiac glycoside andromedotoxin as well as several other toxic substances.
ii. Paroxysmal tachycardia, atrial fibrillation, extra systoles, premature ventricular beats, and ectopic ventricular contractions.
iii. Intravenous atropine sulphate (0.04mg/kg) followed in two minutes with calcium gluconate (2mg/kg by slow i/v injection over the next five minutes). Within 10 minutes, the ECG was almost normal; at 30 minutes, it was entirely normal. At that point, a stomach tube was passed through the oesophagus and into the stomach, and a gastric lavage was performed using only manual restraint. The tortoise made an uneventful recovery.

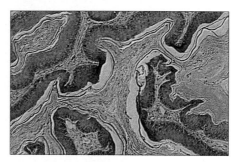

36 i. Epidermal papillomata. Characteristically they are intensely black and proliferative.
ii. Yes, they are infectious between other lizards of this species.
iii. When numerous and/or if they interfere with the affected lizards' eating or other activities, they should be excised. Eventually, most affected lacertid lizards will mount an immune response, and the tumours will regress spontaneously.

The photomicrograph (**above**) shows a histological section. Note the pigmented hyperpigmented dermal extensions. (H & E stain, x67 original magnification).

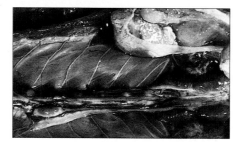

37 ii. Renal portal system. This complex of veins drains the hindlimbs and directs blood partially to the kidneys before it is directed to the liver. Recent investigations have demonstrated that there is a collateral system that bypasses some of this portal circulation, directing a portion of blood from the hindlimbs directly into the hepatic portal flow. Nevertheless, whenever possible, it is advisable to avoid administering potentially toxic drugs into the caudal half of the body. **Above** is a necropsy photomacrograph of a green iguana illustrating the renal portal veins.

38 A mature East African pancake tortoise is presented because of an acute onset of lethargy and tenesmus. A whole-body, dorsoventral radiograph is taken (right).
i. What is your diagnosis?
ii. What would be your immediate management of the case?
iii. What is the most likely cause for this condition?

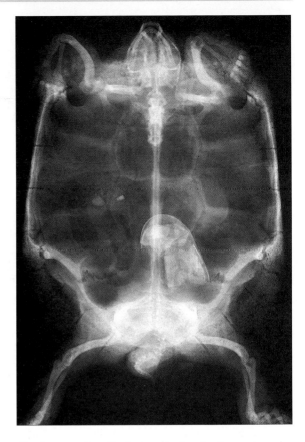

39 One or more intra-oviductal eggs occasionally fracture, thereby lacerating the thin oviduct, and their yolk-rich contents leak into the coelomic cavity of a gravid reptile. This condition can be diagnosed by a variety of investigations including radiographic imaging, fibreoptic laparoscopy, coelomic paracentesis, exfoliative cytology and exploratory celiotomy.
i. What is the clinical significance of this condition?
ii. How would you manage this condition?

40 Giving an enema to reptiles is risky because it may induce an ascending infection involving one or more vital organ systems. Why may this occur in this Class of animals?

41 When attempting to restrain a fractious reptile, why is it inadvisable to use hypothermia to produce anaesthesia?

38 i. Fractured egg in the caudal coelom.
i. Because the sharp edges of the egg point caudally, it is highly unlikely that this egg will be able to pass through the terminal oviduct into the proctodeum and out through the cloaca. Therefore, a coeliotomy and salpingotomy should be performed to remove the broken egg and, if necessary, repair the oviduct.
iii. This type of caudal egg fracture is characteristic of coitus-related damage induced when a sexually aggressive male tortoise mates with a gravid female tortoise; during intromission, the large erect phallus contacts and fractures the egg.

39 i. Egg yolk is extremely reactive and irritating to mesothelial tissues. When intracoelomic tissues are exposed to yolk, an intense cell-mediated inflammatory response called serocoelomitis often occurs.
ii. Egg yolk-induced serocoelomitis must be treated by aggressive surgical intervention comprised of removal of all egg fragments from the coelom, repair of oviductal injuries, and copious lavage and drainage.

40 Reptiles are characterised by having their alimentary and urogenital systems discharge into a common vault-like cloaca rather than through separate body openings. Therefore, introducing fluid into the cloaca carries the risk of transporting pathogenic microorganisms normally present in the cloaca into the postrenal and/or genital tracts and, by doing so, initiating an iatrogenic ascending infection.

41 There is no credible evidence that lowering a reptile's body temperature renders it insensitive to painful stimuli – it only makes it impossible for the creature to react to those stimuli. Even a relatively brief period of hypothermia can substantially diminish both the humeral and cell-mediated immune responses in reptiles whose immune competence is highly temperature-dependent.

42 This 15-year-old red-eared slider turtle had been raised since it was a hatchling on a diet of peeled shrimp and iceberg lettuce. At the time that it was presented for examination, it was not using its hindlimbs; rather, when it was picked up and held vertically, they dangled loosely. The turtle's shell was flat, deformed and markedly soft to the touch.

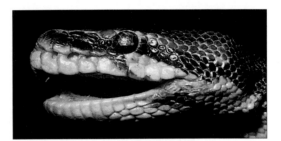

i. What is your tentative diagnosis?
ii. What would you do to confirm your diagnosis?
iii. How would you treat it?

43 This juvenile python exhibits three clinical abnormalities. What are your diagnoses of these three related, but different, disorders?

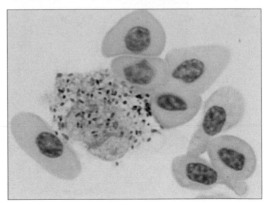

44 The photomicrograph is of a stained blood film from an iguana with multiple chronic abscesses.
i. What are the intracytoplasmic objects within the large, pale-staining cell in the centre of the image?
ii. How does this cell help determine your treatment and prognosis of this case?

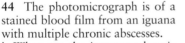

45 Whether or not a complete shelf-like hard palate divides the nasal cavity from the oral cavity is of importance when considering the drinking and other living habits of many reptiles and how a particular reptile must be anaesthetised. In which reptiles does a hard palate divide the oral cavity from the nasal cavities?

42 i. Chronic metabolic bone disease and secondary nutritional hyperparathyroidism due to a calcium-poor, phosphorus-rich diet.
ii. Radiographs revealed a deformed and poorly mineralised skeleton; blood calcium on the day of presentation was 4.6mg/dl.
iii. Calcium gluconate (2.5mg/kg intracoelomically every 48 hours for one week). The diet should be changed immediately to include whole fish, freshly caught earthworms, calcium-rich collard leaves, and algae. Exposure to natural unfiltered sunlight or ultraviolet irradiation; oral vitamin D_3 at a dosage of 1–4 IU/kg twice weekly.

43 (1) Retained tertiary spectacles and dysecdysis – one or more senescent spectacles cover the left eye, and shreds of old epidermis remain unmoulted at the oral commissure and cover the left external nare.
(2) Dyspnoea – the snake is resorting to open-mouth breathing.
(3) Dehydration – the integument is wrinkled and the oral mucosa is dry.

44 i. Phagocytised bacteria.
ii. Although finding engulfed bacteria within circulating leukocytes is evidence of an intact cell-mediated immune response to infection, it also suggests that the organisms responsible for the multiple abscesses have gained entry to the vascular system and are becoming disseminated. Treat aggressively with broad-spectrum bacteriocidal antibiotics and supportive therapy. The prognosis would have been more favourable if evidence of haematogenous spread of infection had not been found.

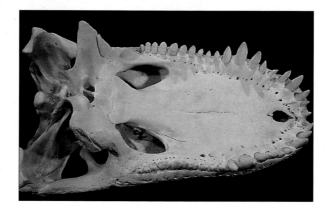

45 Only the crocodilians (crocodiles, alligators, caimans, and gharials). These semi-aquatic animals are able to open their mouths beneath the surface of the water and still inhale and exhale air during respiration. The picture **above** shows an osteological preparation of alligator skull illustrating the complete and solid hard palate that separates the oral and nasal cavities.

46 An indigo snake, a species that feeds upon fish, frogs, small rodents, birds and even other reptiles, is noted during a physical examination to have many small black objects on its oral and pharyngeal mucosa (**right**).
i. What is your diagnosis?
ii. What is the significance of these objects?
iii. How is this condition treated?

47 Reptiles, like fish and amphibians, are thought of as being 'cold-blooded.' Some, however, produce internal body warmth without having to resort to basking in the sun. Which reptiles produce internal body warmth at least during part of their lives?

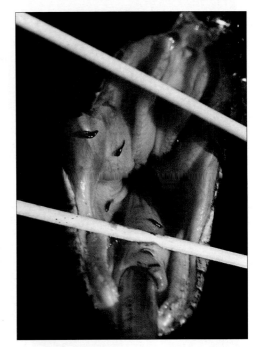

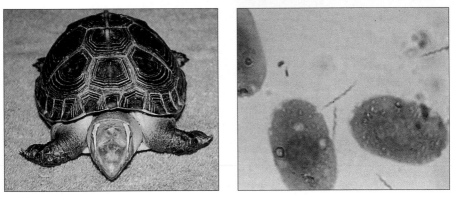

48 This is one of a shipment of Asian box turtles that was received by a pet distributor (**above, left**). Several of these turtles exhibited marked depression and died within a day or two after arrival. Once a diagnosis was made, the rest of the turtles were treated and recovered. A stained blood film (**above, right**) was made from one of these turtles.
i. What is your diagnosis?
ii. What would your treatment be for the rest of the turtles?

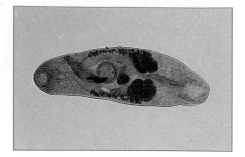

46 i. The black objects are ochetosomid trematodes, one of which has been cleared and mounted (**above**).
ii. While not highly pathogenic, these flukes, when present in large numbers, can cause irritation to the host.
iii. Treatment consists of physically removing the flukes from the oropharynx and cranial oesophagus, and treating the snake with praziquantel (8mg/kg, repeated after two weeks).

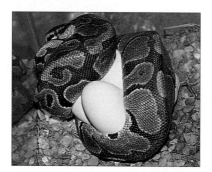

47 Some brooding female pythons, while coiled about their incubating eggs, and, perhaps, some large sea turtles, particularly the leatherback, are two examples of reptiles that are capable of producing significant amounts of endogenous heat by metabolic means. In brooding pythons, heat is produced by rhythmic and periodic muscle-twitching; in leatherback turtles, an efficient countercurrent flow to and from the extremities and, perhaps, a high oil content in the soft tissues contribute to their ability to maintain warmer deep-core body temperatures than the surrounding cold sea. Some very large reptiles, such as adult Komodo and other monitor lizards, crocodilians and, perhaps, some massive turtles, may experience a transient rise in deep-core body temperatures during the digestion of particularly huge meals. **Above** is a brooding royal python and her clutch of eggs.

48 i. Spirochaetosis.
ii. Daily intramuscular injections of enrofloxacin (10mg/kg for 10 days) and daily intracoelomic injections of lactated Ringer's solution (20ml/kg for 10 days).

49 This whole-body dorsal projection radiograph (**right**) is of an adult American bullfrog. What is your diagnosis?

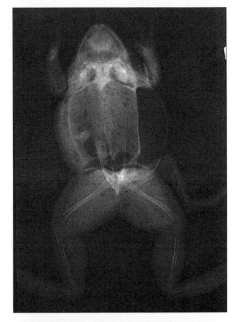

50 Reptiles possess a cloaca through which the faeces, urinary wastes and reproductive products are passed. The eggs or living young pass through which of the following tubular structures on their way out of the gravid female's body?
i. Urodeum.
ii. Urethra.
iii. Copradeum.
iv. Vestibule.
v. Proctodeum.

51 The diet-related disorder steatitis occurs occasionally in captive reptiles, but probably does not occur in wild reptiles eating natural diets. Steatitis is a condition in which body fat becomes chronically inflamed and altered grossly and microscopically. This boa constrictor was fed an abnormal diet which led to its body fat becoming hard and yellow-orange.

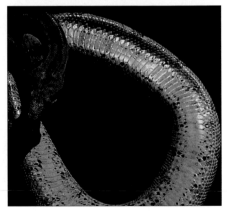

i. What nutritional practices can induce steatitis?
ii. Can steatitis be reversed?
iii. If so, how?
iv. What is the prognosis?

52 Newts and salamanders have become increasingly popular as aquarium pets. Many species of newts and salamanders attain reproductive maturity while retaining their larval external morphology. Thus, although their somatic maturity appears to be delayed, they achieve sexual maturity and can reproduce even though outwardly they still resemble immature gill-bearing larvae. What is the term used to describe the type of development exhibited by these amphibians?

49 Supernumerary left hindlimb.

50 v. Proctodeum.

51 i. Generally, any circumstance that results in the ingestion of high levels of saturated fats or fatty acids can induce steatitis. In this instance, the boa was fed a diet consisting entirely of grossly obese laboratory rats that had been fed an experimental ration consisting of only sunflower seeds and water. As a consequence, the snake received an extremely fat-laden diet.
ii. Yes.
iii. By administering oral or injectable vitamin E (50mg/kg daily) and a change of diet to one which does not contain high levels of lipid.
iv. The prognosis depends largely upon the chronicity: if diagnosed early, this condition is resolved with specific treatment; more chronic disease may be difficult to treat because the lesions may have become isolated by dense fibrocollagenous connective tissue capsules that inhibit the cellular distribution of alpha- and mixed tocopherols.

52 Neoteny. An example of this form of delayed somatic development that is accompanied by sexual maturity is the axolotl (**below**).

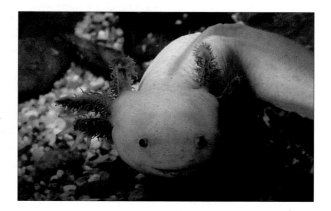

53 This photomicrograph is of a stained blood film from an iguana at x40 magnification.

i. Based upon what you see in this field (which is typical of this specimen), what is your interpretation and tentative diagnosis?

ii. Based solely upon the examination of this stained blood film and knowing the results of a complete white count (26,900/mm^3), how would you treat this iguana?

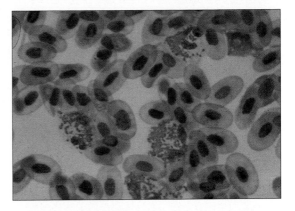

54 i. What is your interpretation of the radiographs (**right**) of this mature iguana?

ii. How would you treat this iguana?

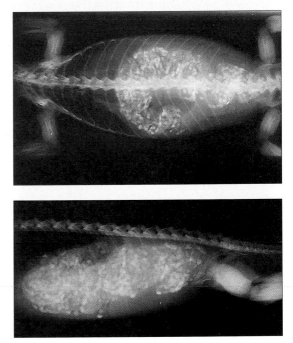

55 Pathogenic bacteria can be transferred from an infected female reptile's ovaries to her eggs before the eggshells are secreted. What important zoonotic pathogen can be transmitted from a female oviparous reptile to her viable eggs?

39

53   i. Leukocytosis in general; heterophilia, specifically.
ii. Broad-spectrum bacteriocidal antibiotic therapy, parenteral fluid therapy and aggressive supportive nursing care.

54   i. Multifocal metabolic bone disease involving the long bones of all four limbs, and the presence of radiopaque foreign bodies throughout the alimentary tract.
ii. This iguana may have been ingesting calcareous material in an effort to obtain the necessary calcium that its diet lacked. Give vitamin D_3 (4iu/kg orally twice weekly), or expose the iguana to unfiltered sunlight or full-spectrum ultraviolet light so that it can synthesise its own vitamin D_3. The diet should be changed to one containing a high level of calcium, a relatively low level of phosphorus and high-quality nutritive fibre. Milk of magnesia, petroleum jelly, or a similar laxative agent, should be given orally to help excretion of the gastrointestinal foreign bodies.

55   *Salmonella* of many serotypes. The species most often cultured is *S. enteritidis*. There are now over 200 serotypes found in reptiles that have been elucidated; many of these are pathogenic for both reptiles and humans.

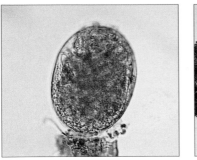
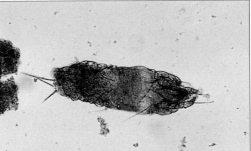

56 These objects (**above**) are found in the faeces of rat snakes.
i. What are they?
ii. Are they clinically significant?

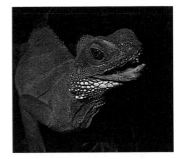

57 The severe rostral abrasions and gingival avulsion seen in this Asian water dragon lizard are frequently encountered, captivity-related conditions and therefore much easier to prevent than to treat.
i. How would you treat these lesions?
ii. How can this kind of rostral and gingival trauma best be prevented?

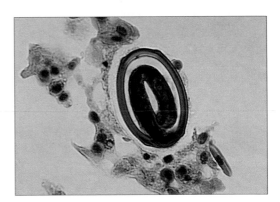

58 This is an example of many oval, thick-shelled objects with small paired projections at each end that were found during a routine faecal examination of the stools from a Savannah monitor lizard.
i. What are these objects?
ii. Are they clinically significant?
iii. If clinically significant, what is an appropriate treatment?

56 i. A mite ovum and a mature mite.
ii. They are not clinically significant because they are mouse parasites. They originated on the fur of the rodent prey that was fed to this snake; hence, they were found in this snake's faeces.

57 i. Exposed and devitalised bone should be excised even though some of the teeth will be lost. The gingiva should be closed over the site where mandibular bone has been lost. Treatment with a topical antibiotic cream or ointment, or an antiseptic plastic wound dressing, will permit lesions such as these to heal more readily.
ii. This lesion is typical of those suffered by reptiles that collide with the solid, transparant walls of their enclosures. Providing a visual barrier often helps prevent this type of trauma because the reptile will be able to see the limits of its habitat and, thus, avoid crashing into the walls of its cage.

58 i. Spiruroid ova.
ii. Yes, these helminth parasites are highly significant.
iii. Ivermectin (200mcg/kg s/c or orally, repeated after two weeks) is an effective treatment for spiruroidiasis in all reptiles except chelonians. Turtles, tortoises and terrapins should not be wormed with ivermectin. Levamisole (5mg/kg i/p, repeated after two weeks) or fenbendazole (50–100mg/kg, repeated after two weeks) is effective in chelonians.

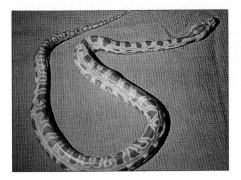
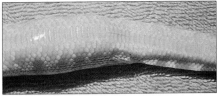

59 A two-month-old amelanistic python (the offspring of sibling parents) developed a steadily expanding bulge just caudal to its umbilical scar (**above**). It had consumed a mouse three weeks earlier, but had refused to accept food thereafter. Yellowish urates had been passed, but faeces had not.

i. What would be your tentative diagnosis?

ii. How would you confirm your diagnosis?

60 Although this young adult male iguana had been growing well on a diet of mixed collard, mustard, turnip, and dandelion greens, and soft ripe fruit, its owner noticed that it was having difficulty eating. On opening the mouth, a firm expansive lesion, distorting the inner surface of the jaw and incarcerating the tongue, so that the iguana could not prehend and swallow items of food, was found arising from the right mandibular ramus.

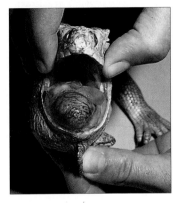

i. What is your diagnosis?

ii. What would be your treatment for this disorder?

iii. What is the prognosis?

iv. How does this case differ from another very common disorder seen in captive iguanas that may share one or more clinical features?

61 In their native habitats, some reptiles (particularly some snakes and large lizards, such as tegus and some monitors) feed on eggs as a major constituent of their diet. However, when these same species of reptiles are fed eggs in captivity, they often develop a biotin deficiency.

i. Why does this disorder occur in captivity, but not in the wild?

ii. How can this nutritional deficiency be prevented in captivity?

59 i. Retained yolk sac; colo-rectal atresia.

ii. Radiography would be useful, but a radiopacity in the region of the mass would not have confirmed the diagnosis. A percutaneous aspiration might have yielded yellow yolk, but often any yolk that has been retained is inspissated and cannot be aspirated. In this case, an exploratory coeliotomy was performed. A complete atresia of the colon and rectum was found and repaired with an end-to-side anastomosis.

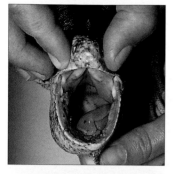

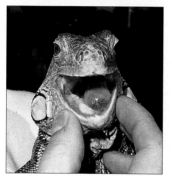

60 i. Ossifying fibroma.

ii. Because the mass was encarcerating the tongue, it should be reduced in size by debulking utilising sharp surgical excision and then applying cryosurgical freezing to the resulting bed of bleeding neoosseous tissue (**left**).

iii. The prognosis is favourable because the condition is often self-limiting.

iv. Ossifying fibromata differ from metabolic bone disease in several aspects: they are often unilateral rather than bilateral; usually, they affect only mandibular bone rather than appendicular long bones; they affect lizards fed nutritious diets that are rich in calcium; and they are histologically distinct from the osseous alterations characteristic of metabolic bone disease.

61 i. Under natural conditions, these reptiles consume **embryonated** eggs rather than infertile eggs which are produced commercially for human consumption. While the albumen portion of the infertile eggs contains avidin, embryonated eggs not only contain much less avidin, but their embryonic tissues also contain biotin.

ii. Vary the diet of these large lizards to include small rodents and fowl chicks. When rodents are being used for prey, they should be given a full meal before being euthanised; thus, the gut contents of these prey will be utilised by the predators. Also, tegus will eat fresh ripe fruit which helps improve the nutritional quality of their diet.

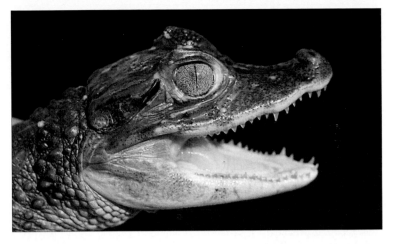

62 This juvenile spectacled caiman is one of several dozen farm-raised animals in a crowded holding pen exhibiting identical lesions with multiple pale grey spots on the integument covering the head, neck, and limbs.
i. What is your diagnosis?
ii. How would you manage this condition in this population of farm-raised animals?
iii. What would you recommend that the caimans' owner do to prevent this from recurring?

63 i. What is your interpretation of this radiograph of a mature female Asian water dragon lizard?
ii. What is the prognosis for this condition?

64 One of the most interesting features of reproductive physiology in reptiles is the storage of viable spermatozoa in some mated females. Consequently, successful males can potentially sire more offspring than if they had to deposit sperm for each ovulatory event in each available female within a population. For how long can this storage last in some snakes, lizards, and chelonians?
i. 2–4 weeks.
ii. 2–4 months.
iii. 2–4 years.
iv. 2–4 hours.
v. 2–4 minutes.

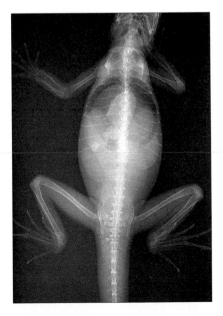

62   i. Caiman pox.
ii. If caimans are being kept in overcrowded enclosures, the population density should be reduced, and great care must be taken to ensure that water quality is maintained at a high level. Topical antiseptics and antibiotics can be used to treat opportunistic bacterial and fungal infections that often take advantage of the already virus-damaged tissues. If some animals are not well enough to eat by themselves, they may have to be fed via a stomach tube. It is important that stress be minimised during the recovery phase of this infection.
iii. A strict quarantine programme must be instituted and adhered to so that newly acquired animals cannot bring disease, previously not present in the colony, into the population at risk. Overcrowding must be avoided, and strict attention to hygiene, food quality and overall husbandry practises is mandatory.

63   i. Gravidity. This lizard has eight shelled eggs in her caudal reproductive tract.
ii. The prognosis is excellent. The skeleton is well mineralised, the eggs are not substantially larger than the mean cross-sectional pelvic diameter, and at least one egg is already positioned within the pelvic outlet and should pass without difficulty.

64   iii. 2–4 years.

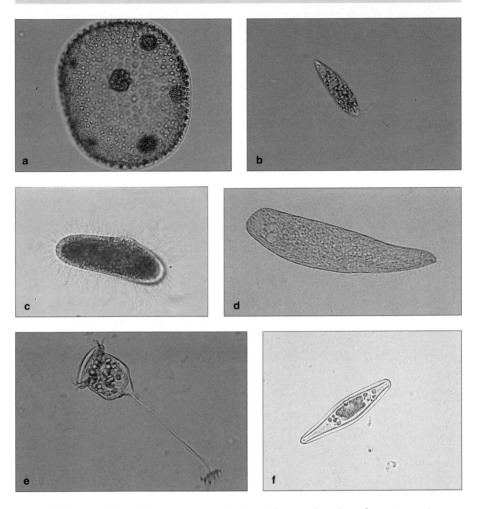

65 While examining the tank water obtained from a breeder of semi-aquatic turtles, these organisms were found.
i. What are these organisms?
ii. Are any of them pathogenic?
iii. If so, which ones?

66 While performing a necropsy on a large snake, you find a greenish cystic structure adjacent to the spleen and pancreas (all are separated from the liver). What is this organ?

65 i. These are commensal protozoan and diatomaceous organisms often found in fresh water. They are:

a: *Volvox.*
b: *Euglena.*
c: *Paramaecium bursaria.*
d: *Blepharoplasma.*
e: *Vorticella.*
f: An unidentified diatom.

ii. None of these freshwater organisms are pathogenic. (Some marine [saltwater] diatoms produce highly virulent toxins that can accumulate in the soft tissues of molluscs.)

66 Gall bladder. Unlike the anatomical placement in other reptiles, a snake's gall bladder is not contiguous with the liver; rather, it joins the pancreas and spleen and is connected to the liver by a long bile duct.

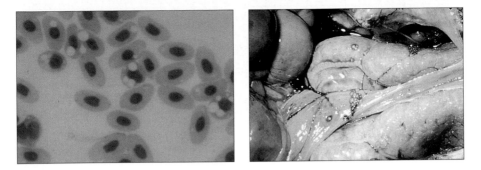

67 An adult male common green iguana was presented for examination showing bilaterally symmetrical caudal coelomic swellings. These masses could be seen as bulges distorting the skin of the belly. They were palpated readily as firm, but slightly yielding, objects that nearly filled the caudal coelom. Repeated blood chemistry investigations over a period of nearly one year had disclosed consistent hyperkalemia and there was a consistent tendency for the blood to haemolyse. The majority of the erythrocytes contained multiple 'punched-out' clear lesions in the haemoglobin (**above, left**). Based upon the presence of this gross haemoglobinopathy (which is consistent with iguana herpesvirus infection), the lizard was treated with a six-week course of oral acyclovir (80mg/kg once daily). Within approximately two weeks, the iguana was eating well and had regained the lost weight. He appeared to be in good health until approximately nine months later at which time abdominal distension was evident and appetite had diminished. Blood was withdrawn from the ventral caudal vein for haematology and clinical chemistry studies (see below).

Examination of a stained specimen of markedly turbid coelomic fluid obtained by paracentesis disclosed a population of bacterial cocci and rods, mixed mononuclear inflammatory leukocytes, and mesothelial cells. Exploratory coeliotomy revealed the symmetrically enlarged organs. A wedge biopsy of one of the enlarged organs was obtained for histopathology, and the coelomic cavity was repeatedly flushed with sterile saline and antibiotic solution. A drain was installed so that daily coelomic lavage could be performed and excess fluid could be removed.

Treatment consisted of oral enrofloxacin (10mg/kg daily), prednisone (2.5mg/kg daily) and intracoelomic injections of sterile physiologic fluid (25ml/kg every 24 hours). The iguana accepted food when it was handfed and made an uneventful recovery.

It appeared to be doing well until the herpesvirus infection recurred 12 days postoperatively; at that time, pharyngeal swelling and dysphagia were noted. Examination of a Wright's-stained blood film disclosed many erythrocytes with 'punched-out' lesions identical to those previously found, a leukocytosis of 26×10^3 WBC/mm^3 and 73% heterophils. The photograph (**above, right**) was taken during necropsy of an iguana which died as a result of this same disorder.

i. What is your diagnosis?

ii. Why were the results of the clinical chemistry investigations not suggestive of the major underlying pathology?

iii. What major clues to the identity of this disorder were suggested by even the earliest physiological chemistry studies?

67 i. Very severe interstitial nephritis and hepatic fibrosis. The iguana was also infected with iguana herpesvirus.

ii. It was not until a substantial amount of both the renal and hepatocellular tissues (and their functions) were destroyed, that clinical chemistry values became abnormal. These organs have a remarkable ability to maintain function well after at least half of their mass has been lost to chronic disease; in cases of acute liver disease, particularly hepatic necrosis, some test results will reflect grossly abnormal enzyme levels. Chronic disease may be masked by the liver's ability to continue to function sufficiently well until late in the course of a disease process.

iii. One of the first clues that caused concern was the finding of many erythrocytes with multiple 'punched-out' clear spaces in their cytoplasm. This lesion is often seen with iguana herpesvirus infection. This iguana experienced two bouts of herpesvirus re-activation and, in each instance, responded well to treatment with acyclovir. In retrospect, a percutaneous renal biopsy would have disclosed the presence of severe interstitial nephritis. Similarly, a liver biopsy would have revealed chronic hepatic fibrosis.

The figure (**below, left**) is a necropsy specimen of a similar case. Note the mottled liver and distended gallbladder. **Below, right** is a low-power photomicrograph of a liver biopsy from a similar case. Note the massive replacement and displacement of the normal hepatocellular architecture by dense fibrous connective tissue. (H & E stain, x27 original magnification).

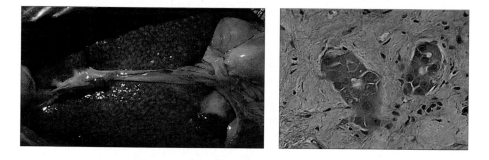

68 What important abnormality is depicted in these erythrocytes?

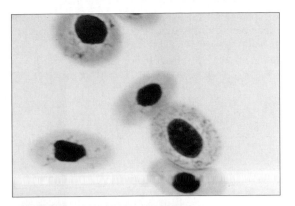

69 A mature female desert tortoise is presented because it has been straining as if to defaecate. A whole-body radiograph is taken.
i. What is your diagnosis?
ii. What would you do to provide relief?

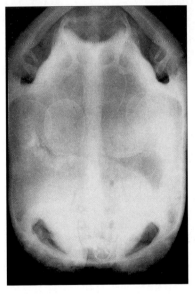

70 The embryonic development and viability of many incubating snake and tortoise eggs can best be monitored during incubation by which of the following methods?
i. Radiographic imaging and lithotripsy.
ii. Auscultation and percussion.
iii. Fibreoptic endoscopy.
iv. Candling and Doppler ultrasonography.
v. Sacrificing an egg from time to time by opening it to examine the contents.

68 Basophilic stippling, highly suggestive of chronic lead toxicosis. Note: new methylene blue stain was applied to a duplicate blood film from this animal and it did not reveal reticulocytosis.

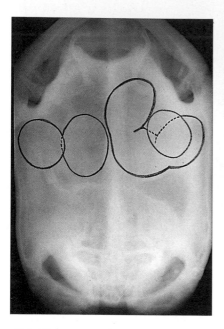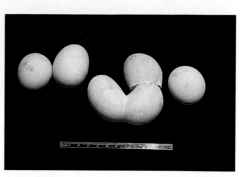

69 i. Three anomalous eggs which share a common eggshell, along with three normal shelled eggs, are present within the oviducts. The same image is enchanced (**above, left**) to better demonstrate the anomalous eggs. The entire clutch of eggs were removed surgically (**above, right**).
ii. Although the three normal eggs could probably pass through the pelvic canal uneventfully, there is no possibility that the three eggs that are united by their conjoined common shells would pass normally. Therefore, they must be removed surgically through a salpingotomy after a transplastral coeliotomy has been performed.

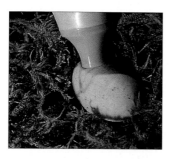

70 iv. Candling and Doppler ultrasonography. The illustration (**left**) shows Doppler ultrasound monitoring of embryonic heart beat and blood flow in an incubating iguana egg.

71 This radiograph (**right**) shows a juvenile water monitor lizard in sternal recumbency.
i. What does the radiograph reveal?
ii. How would you manage this case?

72 Rattlesnakes and Old World vipers are viviparous (they give birth to living young); cobras, mambas, kraits, coral snakes and bushmasters are oviparous (they reproduce by laying eggs).
i. Are the neonates or hatchlings of these snakes dangerous immediately after they are born or hatched?
ii. If not, when do they become venomous?

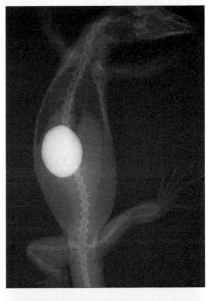

73 i. If you were examining the right eye of this juvenile gecko, what would be your diagnosis?
ii. What should your treatment be for this condition?

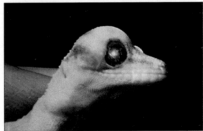

74 Green iguanas are folivores, ie, they are leaf-eating herbivorous lizards. Cellulose is poorly digested until it is processed extensively by gastrointestinal microflora.
i. Where does this intestinal processing of cellulose occur in the iguana?
ii. Where, when and how do iguanas acquire their microflora?

75 Most orders of reptiles have three-chambered hearts – paired atria and a single ventricle; a ridge of myocardial tissue helps direct the blood flow so that the mixing of oxygenated and poorly oxygenated blood is minimised. However, one Order of reptiles has evolved a functional four-chambered heart characterised by anatomically separate right and left ventricles.
i. Which reptiles have a functional four-chambered heart?
ii. Why is this fact clinically significant?

71 i. An ingested radiopaque foreign object, suggestive of a large stone.

ii. The lizard was anaesthetised briefly (oxygen/nitrous oxide/isoflurane mixture using face mask induction) and a Doyen intestinal forceps was inserted into the oesophagus and stomach. The jaws of the forceps were opened and used to grasp and retrieve the smooth stone. The monitor lizard made an uneventful recovery. This case illustrates the enormous size of objects that some reptiles can ingest (and that can be retrieved non-surgically).

72 Yes. The neonates of venomous reptiles are fully capable of producing severe, even fatal, bites; therefore, they must always be handled with great care and respect.

73 i. Periorbital abscess.

ii. Incise and drain the abscess cavity, and flush with 0.75% chlorhexidine solution twice daily until the lesion is healed. Oral antibiotics can be given easily to this partially frugivorous lizard by mixing the drug in with its soft fruit.

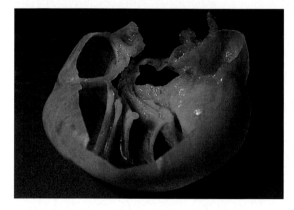

74 i. In the hindgut, specifically in the greatly expanded caecal-colon complex (**left**) which is subdivided into multiple chambers in which fermentation takes place.

ii. Neonatal iguanas acquire their gut microflora shortly after they emerge from their egg chamber beneath the ground; they seek out and consume the freshly deposited faeces of other iguanas.

75 i. Only the crocodilians possess a heart that is anatomically and functionally four-chambered. Chelonian, snake, lizard and sphenodon (Tuatara) hearts are characterised by their two atria and one ventricle. In those reptiles possessing a three-chambered heart, substantial co-mingling of oxygenated and non-oxygenated blood does not occur because the intracardiac blood flow is partially separated by the heart valves, and a ridge of myocardial muscle helps direct the blood flow within the organ.

ii. Because only the crocodilian heart is four-chambered, the sounds produced by intracardiac blood flow and valvular action differ from those of other reptiles. This is particularly evident when employing a Doppler ultrasonic blood flow detector which greatly amplifies the sounds of blood flow.

76 Snakes, unlike almost all other predatory vertebrates, have the ability to swallow enormous-sized prey whole. This is due to the specialised bones of the skull, as illustrated in this Gaboon viper.

i. What are these bones called?
ii. How do they function?

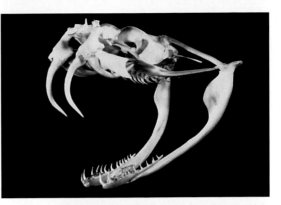

77 This is the right forelimb of a mature female common green iguana that was examined because of a reluctance to place weight upon this leg (right). The previous health history was unremarkable. The diet was collard, mustard, turnip and dandelion greens, fresh ripe fruit and small amounts of firm tofu (soybean curd). The iguana had previously deposited one clutch of eggs, but since she was not kept with a male the infertile eggs had been discarded. Physical examination manifested easily elicited pain when the right carpus was palpated gently. Very loud (VI/VI) systolic and diastolic atrioventricular and aortic valvular murmurs were heard with the aid of an ultrasonic Doppler blood flow detector; these adventitious valvular sounds radiated up the brachiocephalic and carotid arteries and outward through the subclavian arteries. The white blood count was 27,800/mm^3 with a marked left shift, heterophilia and monocytosis. Radiographs disclosed marked osteolysis of the distal right radius and ulna (below, right). The carpal lesion was incised, and a specimen of the material removed was submitted for microbiological culture. What are your tentative diagnoses?

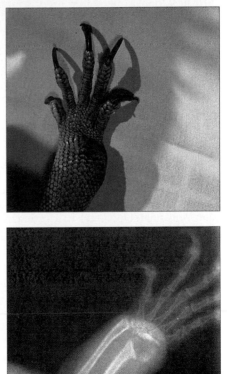

76 i. The quadrate bones.

ii. The quadrate bones are freely suspended and, when rotated forward and downward, they work in concert with the loosely united mandibles and moveable bones of the snout, thus enabling them to stretch widely and accommodate and ingest meals consisting of relatively enormous prey that appear to be too large to be engulfed.

77 Tentative diagnoses include: (1) abscessation; (2) traumatic injury; (3) arthritis; (4) osteomyelitis; (5) metabolic bone disease; (6) non-infectious cyst formation; (7) neoplasia; and (8) subcuticular parasitism. Although there was no fresh evidence of trauma, the soft, painful swelling is suggestive of an infection. However, trauma to either the distal radius and ulna and/or the carpal joint cannot be discounted. Arthritis is possible, but no other joints were involved. A cyst or a neoplasm arising from the joint capsule or synovial membrane is a possible, although less likely, diagnosis as is the presence of a subcutaneous parasite. Several clues were given in the details of the diet, the Doppler blood-flow investigation findings, the haematology results and the radiographs.

The iguana had been on an appropriate high-calcium, low-phosphorus, good-quality leafy vegetable diet. The Doppler instrument detected loud valvular murmurs that radiated outward from their origins. The WBC was entirely consistent with a severe bacterial infection. Radiography disclosed a severely osteolytic process that was destroying the distal ends of the ulna and carpus; a culture taken from a specimen of exudate aspirated from the distal forelimb yielded *Salmonella urbana, Staphylococcus aureus,* beta-haemolytic *Streptococcus*, and an *Enterococcus*.

Euthanasia was carried out and a necropsy performed. The distal limb lesion evinced severe pyogranulomatous osteitis and arthritis. When the heart was opened, every valve was found to be involved in vegetative endocarditis (**below**). *Salmonella urbana* and the same beta-haemolytic *Streptococcus* were cultured from several fragmented mural thrombi attached to the atrio-ventricular and aortic heart valves. Multiple visceral organs were found with abscesses that yielded the identical *Salmonella* and beta-haemolytic *Streptococcus*. Microthromboemboli were found in numerous small blood vessels. The final diagnosis was osteomyelitis and septic arthritis with secondary disseminated bacterial vegetative endocarditis, endocardiosis, and thromboembolism.

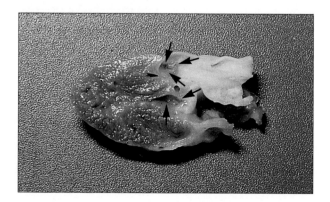

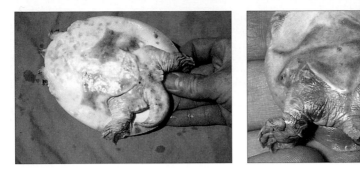

78 This is a soft-shelled turtle with integumentary lesions (**above, left**) and another with more advanced disease (**above, right**).
i. What is the significance of the red lesions scattered randomly over the plastral integument of each turtle?
ii. What is the aetiology of this condition?
iii. How is this condition treated?

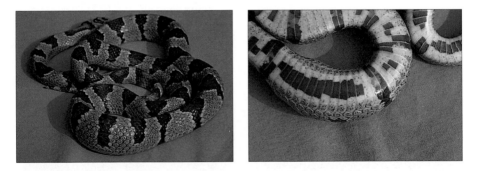

79 A North American banded king snake is presented because, although the snake has a hearty appetite, it has regurgitated each rodent meal undigested within 24–36 hours after swallowing. Physical examination discloses an active, well-fleshed snake whose only grossly observable abnormality is a swelling in the region of the stomach (**above**).
i. What is your tentative diagnosis?
ii. What specific test(s) should be carried out to help confirm your diagnosis?
iii. What is the prognosis?
iv. What are your recommendations to the owner to prevent this condition?

78 i. The turtle on the **left** shows early lesions of septicemic cutaneous ulcerative disease (SCUD); that on the **right** is a more advanced case. Note the crateriform lesions filled with necrotic debris.

ii. The aetiologic agent of SCUD is *Citrobacter freundii*.

iii. This disease can be treated effectively with almost any bacteriocidal antibiotic together with supportive nursing care. Presently, enrofloxacin (10mg/kg daily i/m or orally) is effective.

79 i. Cryptosporidiosis.

ii. Gastric lavage, concentrating the fluid recovered, treating it with acid-fast stain, and examining the specimen microscopically for the presence of *Cryptosporidium serpentis* (**below, left**). A biopsy of the gastric mucosa also can be obtained by using a gastroscope. The photomicrograph (**below, right**) is of such a gastric biopsy. Note the myriad number of organisms attached to the luminal mucosal epithelial cells lining the gastric pits.

iii. The prognosis is very guarded. Currently, there are no effective treatments known for cryptosporidiosis in snakes. Although spiromycin therapy is effective in humans infected with cryptosporidiosis, this drug is not effectual in snakes.

iv. Any snakes that are confirmed to be infected should be destroyed. No snake from this collection should be transferred to another collection. The cages(s) used to house any snakes should be discarded or thoroughly disinfected by treating with live steam, gluaraldehyde, formaldehyde or another powerful disinfectant.

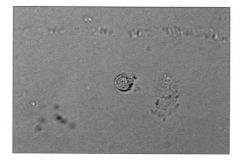 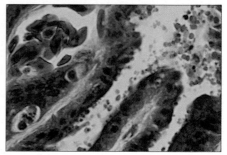

80 This half-grown female common green iguana has a white crystalline substance adhering to the skin surrounding her nostrils.
i. What is this substance?
ii. What is its significance?

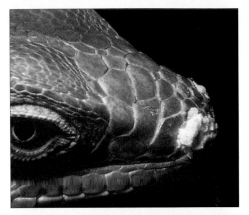

81 Two ova are seen while performing a faecal analysis on a specimen from a Nile monitor lizard.
i. What is your diagnosis?
ii. Are the adult organisms that produced these eggs pathogenic to the lizard?

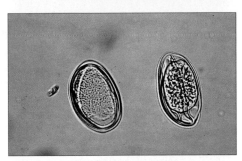

82 This is one of a group of approximately 100 African clawed frogs used in biomedical research that experienced a sudden mortality following a single feeding of thawed, frozen salmon brought into the laboratory by an animal caretaker who had caught the fish. All of the dead and dying frogs shared identical gross lesions consisting of full-thickness cutaneous ulcerations. The mucous integument that surrounded each ulcer was raised and erythematous. Gross necropsy and histopathologic findings were minimal, consisting only of ulceration and mild mononuclear leukocytic infiltration of the denuded skeletal muscle.
i. What is your tentative diagnosis?
ii. What tests would you perform to confirm your diagnosis?

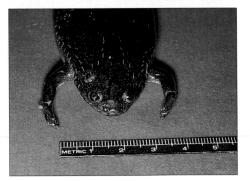

iii. What is the prognosis?
iv. How would you treat the remaining frogs?
v. What control measures should be instituted to prevent a repetition of this problem?

80 i. Salt; sodium chloride and potassium chloride crystals.

ii. Many reptiles possess salt-secreting glands that are located beneath their nasal mucosa (some snakes have sublingual salt glands, and some crocodilians have salt-secreting glands that are imbedded in their tongue). This type of salt secretion is a means by which reptiles discard excess electrolytes (as Na^+, K^+ and Cl^- salts) without the loss of a substantial amount of water and, thus, is a method of water conservation. It is particularly well developed in marine and desert-dwelling reptiles, but is also present in many other reptiles.

81 i. Pentastomiasis. These two ova are from the pentastomid parasite, *Raillietiella* sp.
ii. Yes.

82 i. Aeromoniasis, although similar lesions are seen in other Gram-negative infections.
ii. Microbiological culture, particularly one that is carried out on specimens subcultured in thioglycholate broth and incubated at 30°C and at a reduced oxygen atmosphere.
iii. The prognosis is poor to guarded because of the virulent pathogenicity of many Gram-negative microorganisms in amphibians.
iv. Frogs exposed to this frog and other sick frogs should be isolated and kept in uncrowded treatment tanks. An appropriate bacteriocidal antibiotic, determined by sensitivity testing, should be administered by the intramuscular or oral route; alternatively, enrofloxacin has been shown recently to be effective when added to the tank water in which the frogs under treatment are being kept.
v. Outbreaks such as this one can usually be avoided by adhering to strict quarantine, enhancing sanitary and other hygienic practices, and controlling the food sources. In this instance, the aetiologic agent responsible for the outbreak was *Aeromonas salmonicida*, a common pathogen of salmonid fishes (salmon and trout).

83 An adult female turtle has been regurgitating recently swallowed meals.
i. What was the precipitating factor and what does the radiograph reveal?
ii. What would your treatment be for this turtle?
iii. What is the prognosis?

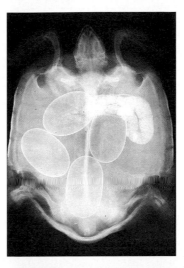

84 A Colombian boa constrictor was treated by its physician owner for ulcerative stomatitis ('mouth rot') with daily injections of streptomycin. After two weeks the snake had not improved, so the owner changed the antibiotic therapy to daily injections of gentamicin, but the snake's condition deteriorated even further. After a further week the owner changed the antibiotic to injectable amikacin given once every 24 hours. Three days after this treatment began, the snake was found dead in its cage. Necropsy examination revealed myriad pale grey to pink nodular lesions within the oral cavity (**above, right**). The kidneys and liver were pale tan and cut with resistance; the pericardial sac was filled with a deposit of white material that adhered to the epicardium; the renal tissues contained 'starburst'-like granulomatous lesions (**below, right**).

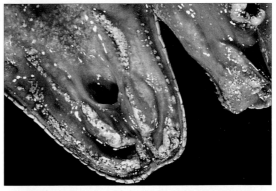

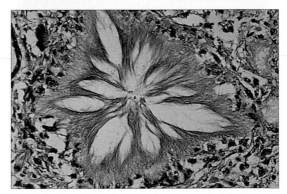

i. What is your diagnosis?
ii. What part of the owner's therapy contributed to this condition?
iii. How could it have been prevented?

83 i. The barium meal study shows the presence of four large shelled eggs, one of which is impinging upon the small intestine.

ii. The shells of each of these eggs is sufficiently mineralised to permit induced deposition using oxytocin. The tortoise should be primed with an initial intracoelomic injection of 10% calcium gluconate, followed in two hours by an intramuscular injection of oxytocin (2 units/100g bodyweight without subtracting the estimated weight of the caparace and plastron).

iii. The prognosis is favourable because as soon as the eggs have been deposited, the extramural pressure on the intestine will be removed.

84 i. Hyperuricaemia and visceral gout.

ii. Each of the antibiotics that was chosen is an aminoglycoside and, therefore, is potentially nephrotoxic. Fluid therapy to maintain safe levels of plasma volume was not given. As each antibiotic was used and abandoned, another was chosen with little or no thought given to the cumulative effects of the entire series.

iii. At no time was there an attempt to submit specimens for microbiological culturing and antibiotic sensitivity testing. The owner merely assumed that the snake would respond to the antibiotics that were administered. Part of any rational protocol of treatment should include the parenteral administration of adequate physiological fluids and electrolytes, provision of additional warmth, and general supportive nursing care.

85 What ophthalmic condition is affecting the right eye of this American alligator?

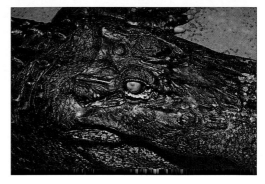

86 A box turtle has sustained a fracture to its carapace several months prior to the date of its examination. During inspection of the turtle, a white cottony substance is noted growing within the shell defect where a piece of shell has been lost (**below, left**). A small specimen of this substance is examined microscopically and is found to contain elongated structures that are divided into two or more compartments (**below, right**).
i. What is your diagnosis?
ii. How is this condition treated?

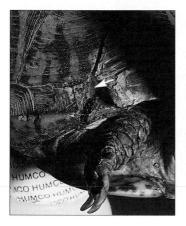
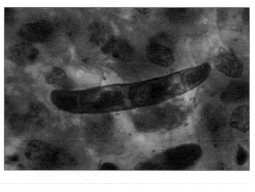

87 Which organ system serves a secondary purpose as a hydrostatic organ in diving reptiles?

85 Post-traumatic corneal pannus and vitiligo (pigment loss) of the eyelids.

86 i. *Microsporum* infection. In this instance, probably an opportunistic infection of the soft tissues that were exposed when the carapace was fractured.
ii. Cleanse the wound thoroughly; treat with a topical fungicide; and give ketoconazole (30mg/kg daily for at least 30 days).

87 The lungs serve as hydrostatic organs as well as respiratory gas-exchange structures (**below**). When the lungs are inflated, the animal can float to the surface; when the lungs are emptied, the animals become negatively buoyant and are therefore able to stay submerged with little effort. Even fully terrestrial chelonians and many lizards retain the ancient pattern in which the lungs continue caudally into the coelomic cavity.

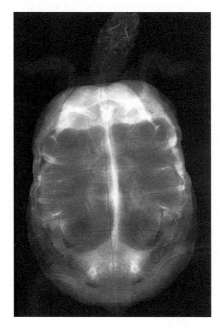

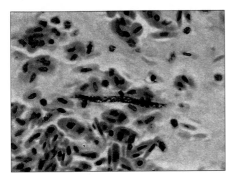 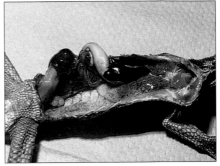

88 These elongated dark organisms (**above, left**) are found in the blood of an East African Fischer's chameleon. The adult forms of similar organisms are embedded within the mesenteries of a helmeted lizard (**above, right**).
i. What are the organisms?
ii. What is their significance?
iii. How would you treat a reptile in which these organisms are detected?
iv. What measures would you take to prevent reinfection from occurring?

89 The skin of the hindlimbs and tail of this juvenile chameleon (**right**) has been severely and repeatedly traumatised; it is one of several kept in a terrarium furnished with artificial plants. The chameleons are offered water *ad libitum* via an overhead drip system and are fed on small crickets.
i. What is your diagnosis?
ii. How can this be prevented?

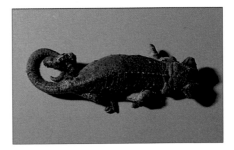

90 An adult female Mexican dwarf 'python' has four large swellings in the caudal half of its body and several deeply indented creases in its body wall. When palpated, these swellings are markedly firm and only minimally mobile within the body cavity. Which of the following combinations are likely diagnoses of this condition?
i. Gastric cryptosporidiosis and pulmonary emphysema.
ii. Hepatic cyst or tumour and gallstone(s).
iii. Urolithiasis, splenomegaly and pancreatic mass.
iv. Cardiomyopathy and oesophageal dilatation.
v. Retained ova and dystocia.

88 i. Microfilariae.
ii. If present in sufficient numbers, microfilariae can obstruct capillaries, venules and sinusoids, thus causing local anoxia and necrosis.
iii. A non-chelonian reptile infected with filarid helminths and their microfilariae offspring can be treated with ivermectin (200mcg/kg, repeated after two weeks). Levamisol can be used in chelonians (5mg/kg by intracoelomic injection, repeated after two weeks).
iv. Like other filarid parasites, these organisms are transmitted by arthropod vectors. Therefore, reptile cages should be screened to prevent entry by haematophagous arthropods, eg, mosquitoes. Vigorous control of mite and tick infestation is also necessary. A sound quarantine programme is essential to reduce the introduction of new disease agents into a collection or colony of reptiles.

89 i. Cricket-induced trauma.
ii. Live crickets fed to captive amphibians and reptiles must be furnished with a source of food so that if they are not immediately consumed as prey, they will have something to eat besides their erstwhile predators.

90 v. This python has four necrotic eggs retained within her oviducts. Gastric cryptosporidiosis, pulmonary emphysema, hepatic cyst, tumour, gallstones, splenomegaly, pancreatic mass, cardiomyopathy, and oesophageal dilatation would not be lesions affecting organs in the caudal half of the body. Urolithiasis is highly unlikely because snakes lack a urinary bladder.

91 This is an unstained wet mount made from the faeces of a Colombian boa constrictor with a history of bloody and mucoid stools (**right**).
i. What are the five organisms shown?
ii. How do these organisms differ?
iii. What is your diagnosis?
iv. What is the prognosis?
v. How would you treat this condition?

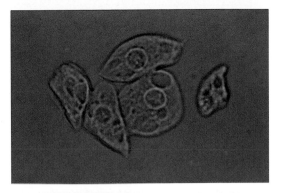

92 During the necropsy of an adult African leopard tortoise, this piece of liver tissue was found. When placed into formalin solution for preservation, it did not sink.
i. What is your interpretation of this liver tissue?
ii. What common husbandry practice is likely to have induced the changes found in the liver of this tortoise?

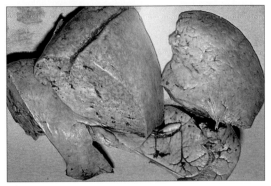

93 A gravid female snake, lizard, or tortoise occasionally experiences difficulty in passing her ova even though radiographs do not reveal abnormalities and a suitable nesting site with appropriate incubation medium is provided. Which of the following should you do in order to aid in the passage of these eggs?
i. Inject calcitonin and oxytocin (or vasotocin) intramuscularly.
ii. Inject testosterone and oxytocin (or vasotocin) intramuscularly.
iii. Inject vitamin D_3 and oxytocin (or vasotocin) intramuscularly.
iv. Inject calcium and oxytocin (or vasotocin) intramuscularly.

91 i. Protozoa.

ii. There are four uninuclear trophozoites and one quadrinuclear cyst.

iii. *Entamoeba invadens.*

iv. The prognosis depends upon the severity of the infection and the amount of damage incurred by the liver and intestines. If diagnosed early and treated aggressively, the prognosis is favourable.

v. Treatment for entamoebiasis is metronidazole (40–250mg/kg depending upon the family of snake being treated: colubrid snakes – 40 mg/kg, repeated after two weeks: Boidae, Viperidae and Elapidae – 125–250mg/kg, repeated after two weeks). Because snakes infected with *Entamoeba invadens* are often profoundly ill and quite labile patients, it is essential to provide antibiotic therapy, fluid replacement and compassionate supportive nursing care in order to achieve a successful resolution of this serious protozoan infection.

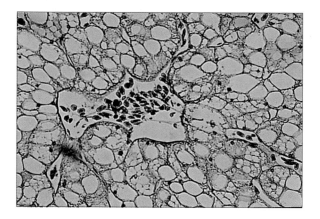

92 i. The liver tissue is heavily infiltrated with fat (**above**).

ii. Fatty infiltration of the liver can be induced by numerous metabolic, toxic and some infectious causes. Most often, this alteration of liver is caused by diets rich in readily available dietary fats, eg, commercial dog, cat and primate food. Most tortoises are facultative herbivores and, thus, thrive on a diet of high-quality nutritive vegetable fibre.

93 iv. Inject calcium and oxytocin (or vasotocin) intramuscularly.

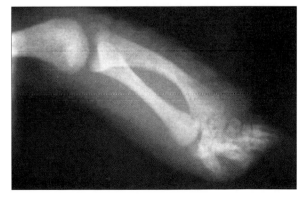

94 This clutch of neonate desert tortoises (**above, left**), was brought to the veterinary surgery by their concerned owner. Each of the baby tortoises had identical developmental anomalies consisting of bilateral anophthalmia, complete forelimb and tail agenesis, maxillofacial clefts, and carapacial, plastral plate and scute abnormalities (**above, right**). The parents of these sibling hatchlings were unrelated and had produced a previous clutch of normal offspring. The only difference noted by the owner between the two clutches of eggs was the means and duration of their incubation. The normal eggs had been incubated in slightly dampened sand kept warm by a heating pad; the abnormal clutch had been incubated in an electric skillet kept on its lowest setting. The eggs from the normal clutch began to hatch on the 121st day of incubation; those from the abnormal clutch began to hatch on the 93rd day of incubation.
i. What is your diagnosis?
ii. What is the aetiology of these anomalies?

95 i. What is your interpretation of this radiograph of the forelimb of a gopher tortoise ?
ii. How would you treat this condition?

96 When suturing reptilian skin, the veterinary surgeon must attempt to produce a slight eversion of the edges of the incision. Why is this manoeuvre necessary?

94 i. Epigenetic (non-heritable) developmental anomalies.
ii. An incubation temperature that was abnormally high induced the nearly identical birth defects in these tortoises. The unusually warm temperature hastened their development and reduced their overall incubation times but, in doing so, resulted in profound skeletal and other deformities.

95 i. Osteochondritis. Several small 'joint mice' can be seen within the ulnocarpal joint space.
ii. Other than surgical exploration of the affected joint and removal of any dislodged bone or cartilage fragments, this joint can be injected aseptically with a small volume of corticosteroid. Aspirin (0.5–1.0mg/kg) might relieve the pain.

Surgery was not performed in this case; rather, a daily dose of 0.50mg/kg (children's) aspirin was given for a period of six weeks; the owners were instructed to report any gross evidence of blood in the tortoise's stools immediately. At six weeks the tortoise exhibited marked and steady improvement and began to use the affected forelimb. The owners of this tortoise were then instructed to reduce the dosage of aspirin to 0.25mg/kg every 48 hrs. The last time this patient was seen was approximately two years after its initial presentation; at that time, it was walking normally. However, radiographically, the lesions were unchanged.

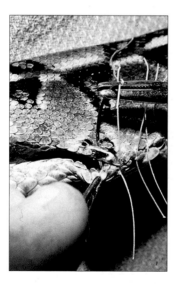

96 Reptilian skin has a tendency to roll inward when incised (mainly due to the abundant subcuticular skeletal muscles that are present). When suturing the integument, the surgeon should appose incisions with a slightly everting pattern so as to bring the incised edges into intimate contact with each other (**left**). Cosmetically attractive healing results from this technique.

97 This photograph was taken during the preliminary examination of the carcase of a royal python. Numerous raised, red lesions are scattered over the inner surfaces of the coelomic cavity.
i. What is your diagnosis of this disorder?
ii. To what nutritional condition are these lesions attributable?
iii. Is this an acute or a chronic condition?

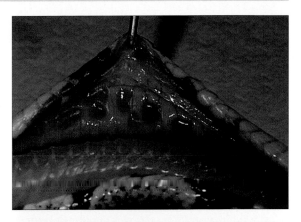

98 The remains of a parasitic ovum from a giant blue-tongued skink are shown.
i. What type of egg is it?
ii. What kind of life cycle does this parasitic organism have?
iii. Is this likely to be pathogenic for a skink?
iv. If pathogenic, what is an appropriate treatment?

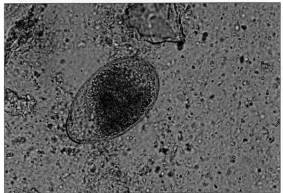

99 i. What are your diagnoses of the conditions afflicting this long-term captive emydid semi-aquatic turtle?
ii. How would you treat this turtle?
iii. What recommendations would you give to the turtle's owner to help prevent these conditions?

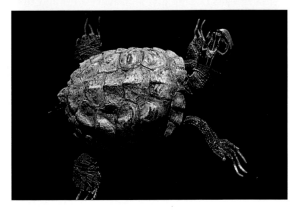

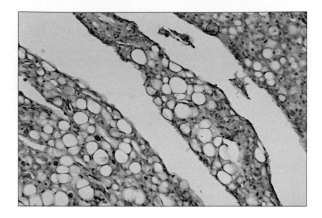

97 i. Serous atrophy of coelomic adipose tissue. Note the cellular fibrous replacement of the usually cell-poor fat body (**above**).
ii. Starvation.
iii. Chronic.

98 i. A trematode.
ii. Flukes utilise a complicated indirect life cycle in which at least one mollusc serves as an intermediate host.
iii. Yes. Finding trematode ova in the stools of skink is consistent with a potentially pathogenic infestation.
iv. Trematodiasis is treated most effectively by parenteral injection of praziquantel (8mg/kg, repeated after two weeks). Although praziquantel can be administered orally, it is most effective when given intramuscularly because many trematodes found in reptilian hosts occupy non-alimentary sites and tissues that are best approached via their vascular supply.

99 i. Overgrowth of the keratinous mouthparts, claws and carapacial shell scutes.
ii. The overgrown mouthparts and claws should be trimmed, and any loosened, but still attached, scutes should be lifted from the underlying plates.
iii. Provide a more natural captive habitat furnished with mildly abrasive surfaces upon which the turtle can wear down its ever-growing keratinous mouthparts and claws. Inspect the turtle periodically and remove the loose, but retained, shell scutes.

100 A sexually mature female corn snake is presented for evaluation because of regurgitation and weight loss. As part of the examination, a radiograph of her mid-body is made.
i. What is your tentative diagnosis?
ii. How would you confirm your diagnosis?

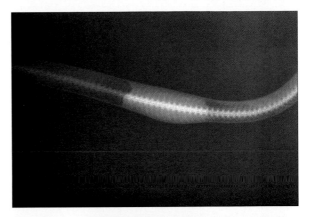

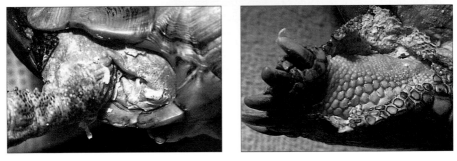

101 This tortoise (**above, left and right**) had had a mild respiratory infection. Microbiological culture and antibiotic sensitivity testing revealed a pure culture of *Pasteurella testudinis* that was highly sensitive to enrofloxacin. The tortoise was treated for 10 days with oral enrofloxacin (10mg/kg). On the first day of treatment, vitamin A was injected intramuscularly into its right foreleg. Supportive therapy consisted of daily injections of intracoelomic fluids (20ml/kg), daily hand feeding of fresh green vegetables and soft fruits, and maintenance at a hospital cage temperature of 34°C. Fourteen days after it was first examined and treated, the skin covering the tortoise's limbs, cervical region and tail became erythematous and swollen. Within two more days large multiple blisters had formed and within another day the affected integument was sloughing away from the underlying skeletal muscles.
i. What is your diagnosis?
ii. What was the aetiology of this condition?
iii. How would you treat this disorder?
iv. What is the prognosis for recovery?
v. How would you avoid a repetition of this condition?

100 & 101: Answers

100 i. Mid-body, fluid-density mass consistent with diffuse gastric hypertrophy; these characteristics are consistent with cryptosporidiosis.
ii. Perform a gastric lavage by passing a plastic or rubber urethral catheter via the oesophagus into the stomach and introduce 5–10ml of lactated Ringer's solution; 'flutter' the now slightly distended stomach briefly with your fingers; withdraw some of the lavage fluid; place a small amount of the fluid on a slide; stain the wet mount with merthiolate, or prepare an acid-fast-stained dry mount; and examine microscopically for the presence of *Cryptosporidium serpentis*.

101 i. Necrotising dermatitis.
ii. Iatrogenic hypervitaminosis A. This condition often follows the intramuscular injection of vitamin A-containing medications. Typically, erythema and early bulla formation are seen approximately 10–12 days after an intramuscular injection of vitamin A. Within a few days, the affected epidermis begins to slough, leaving the subjacent bed of tissue denuded and prone to attack by opportunistic pathogens.
iii. These denuded sites must be cleansed gently and covered with a suitable antibiotic ointment or cream. Parenteral or oral antibiotic therapy is usually indicated, and supportive nursing care to maintain fluid balance, nutrition and environmental warmth is essential.
iv. Favourable. Most affected chelonians make an uneventful recovery.
v. This condition is preventable if vitamin A-containing drugs are used only when there are clinically justifiable reasons for their use; it is best to use an oral form rather an injectable form of vitamin A.

102 A photomicrograph of a stained blood film from a red-eared slider turtle is shown.
i. What is your diagnosis?
ii. What is the significance of this condition?
iii. How would you treat this disorder?

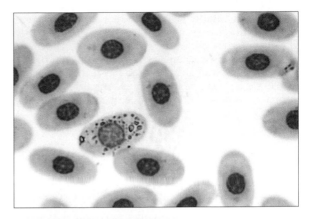

103 This leopard gecko exhibits typical gross lesions of metabolic bone disease. This disorder of osseous mineralisation is relatively common in both herbivorous as well as insectivorous lizards kept in captivity.
i. What can cause this disorder?
ii. What factors should you discuss with the owner?

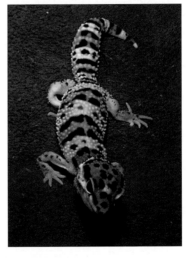

104 Sometimes an herbivorous lizard, eg, a green iguana, is found during necropsy to have skeletal and/or myocardial muscle tissue that is characterised by white or greyish streaks. Which of the following is the most likely combination of deficiencies that is associated with these lesions?
i. Vitamin K and coumadin.
ii. Vitamin D and phosphorus.
iii. Vitamin D and calcium.
iv. Vitamin E and selenium.
v. Vitamin A and phospholipids.

102 i. Plasmodiosis. The refracticle inclusions are intracytoplasmic *Plasmodium* sp.
ii. The major significance of this malarial infection is the potential for anaemia and the over-recruitment of thrombocytes to transform into erythrocytes to make up the deficit in erythrocyte mass; once the thrombocytes are diminished to a threshold level, blood clotting may be inhibited, leading to spontaneous haemorrhage.
iii. Give a 'loading' oral dose of chloroquine phosphate (5mg/kg) and an oral dose of primaquine phosphate (0.5mg/kg); then weekly doses of 2.5mg/kg and 0.5mg/kg respectively for the next three to four months.

103 i. Oversupplementation with vitamin-mineral products can induce iatrogenic hypervitaminosis A and hypervitaminosis D_3 resulting in some forms of metabolic bone disease.
ii. Feed a more natural, well balanced diet so that vitamin-mineral supplementation is not required. Leopard geckos are insectivorous; however, they will consume fruit and soft vegetables avidly as well. Insect prey can be fed beta carotene-rich fresh green, orange and yellow vegetables so that when they are given as prey to the lizards, their beta carotene-rich gut contents will supply the substrate from which vitamin A is synthesised by the geckos. Unfiltered sunlight or a source of unfiltered ultraviolet light will enable the lizards to synthesise vitamin D_3 endogenously.

104 iv. Vitamin E and selenium defeciency can cause 'white muscle' disease. The photomicrograph (**below**) is a histological section of skeletal muscle from a spiny-tailed iguana. Note the pallor, loss of cross-striations, and infiltration by small mononuclear leucocytes (H & E, x67 original magnification).

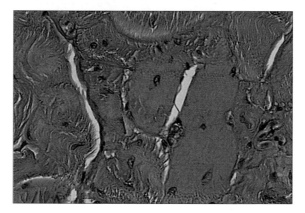

105 A juvenile agama lizard has a swollen left eye.
i. What tests or procedures would you employ to make an accurate diagnosis of this condition?
ii. How would you treat it?

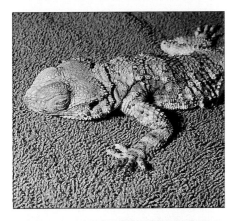

106 These two pairs of organisms joined by thin strands were found in the faeces of a California king snake.
i. What is your diagnosis?
ii. Is this pathogenic?
iii. If pathogenic, what is your treatment?

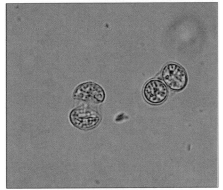

107 The whole-body radiograph (**right**) shows a Pacific pond turtle that has swallowed a fish hook attached to a nylon leader.
i. How would you remove this fish hook and what other treatment is appropriate for this turtle before it is released?
ii. What are some of the postoperative complications that should be considered?

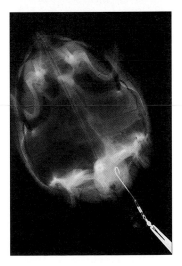

108 What causes the eggshells of some lizards and chelonians to be overly soft when they are deposited?

105 i. Aspirate a sample of exudate for microbiological culture, sensitivity testing, and cytology; apply Gram and PAS stains to obtain a preliminary idea of what bacterial or mycotic pathogens are present.
ii. Incise and drain the swelling, then flush with dilute chlorhexidine solution. Commence oral antibiotic therapy using a broad-spectrum bacteriocidal drug shown to be effective against the general class of pathogen(s) found during examination of the Gram-stained specimen; if necessary, change the antibiotic if the sensitivity testing reveals that the pathogen is resistant to the first drug.

106 i. *Sarcocystis.*
ii. It is not pathogenic to this host; rather, it is pathogenic in its intermediate rodent hosts.
iii. Although treatment is not necessary, a course of trimethoprim-sulphadiazine or trimethoprim-sulphamethoxazole (10–20mg/kg daily for two weeks) is effective in eradicating these protozoa.

107 i. Anaesthetise the turtle so that its mouth can be kept open without it struggling; insert an endoscope or long, narrow speculum over the leader that is still attached to the fishhook; grasp the hook and carefully incise the oesophagus taking care to create as small an incision as possible; retrieve the hook; close the oesophageal wound using buried sutures. Commence a course of bacteriocidal broad-spectrum antibiotic therapy and fluid replacement.
ii. Oesophagitis, oesophageal stricture/stenosis, and oesophageal abscess.

108 The eggshells of most snakes and many lizards are normally rather soft and leathery, and they often swell to accommodate the developing embryo or fetus within. However, the eggshells of most chelonians and crocodilians are usually calcareous. The eggshells of most reptiles will become unnaturally soft under conditions of low dietary calcium intake or hypovitaminosis D_3. Any aetiology that would induce hypocalcaemia, such as primary hypoparathyroidism, can also induce eggshell softening.

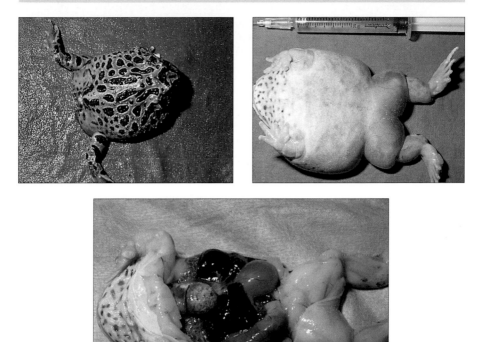

109 This adult male Argentine horned frog (**top, left** and **right**) was examined because it had displayed marked depression and had massive distention of its coelomic cavity. The frog had previously been healthy and had been fed three to five small 'feeder' comet goldfish weighing 9–12g three times weekly. The fish were fed a commercial flaked fish food. The fluid distended not only the coelomic cavity, but had also infiltrated the subcutaneous tissues of the hindlimbs and trunk. When aspirated with a sterile needle the fluid was strongly positive for blood urea nitrogen, had a specific gravity of 1.007, was cell-free and failed to clot even after 10 hours. 18ml of fluid were aspirated, after which the frog exhibited immediate relief, but died four hours later. An additional 8.4ml of fluid was then aspirated. Gross pathology revealed a pericardial sac distended with solid yellow deposits which completely covered and adhered to the epicardium (**above**). The liver was pale brown and had rounded edges. A solitary pale yellow nodule was located where the right and left hepatic lobes joined. The kidneys were slightly enlarged and mottled with minute greyish-yellow foci. A 0.4cm pale yellow urinary calculus was found within the fundus of the urinary bladder. The remaining organs were unremarkable.
i. What is your diagnosis?
ii. How is this condition related to the frog's diet?

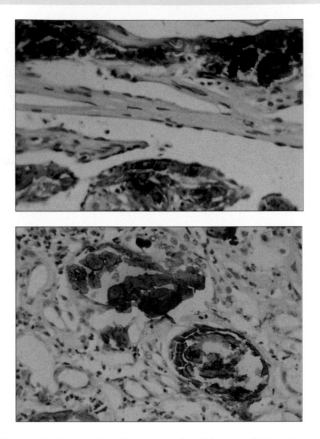

109 i. Multifocal soft-tissue mineralisation and multi-organ failure due to hypervitaminosis D_3 and hypercalcaemia.

ii. The frog acquired enormous dosages of vitamin D_3 when it consumed comet gold-fish that had been fed a commercial flaked fish food just before being eaten by the frog. The hypervitaminosis D_3 favoured an increased uptake of calcium from the large intestine which, in turn, induced the deposition of calcium salts in organ sites not usually calcified. These sites included the heart (**top**), kidneys, liver (**above**), and alimentary tract. Thus, the ascitic fluid probably was related directly or indirectly to: (1) heart failure; (2) renal failure; (3) hepatic failure; and (4) at least a moderate pro-tein-wasting enteropathy. All of these conditions contributed to the accumulation of ascitic and oedema fluid.

110 The cadaver of a common green iguana is shown just prior to its necropsy.
i. What major abnormality does the iguana exhibit?
ii. What visceral organ dysfunction is likely to be involved in this condition?

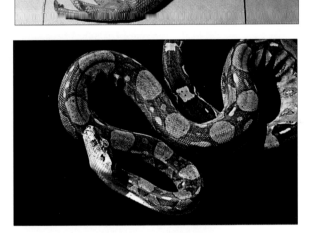

111 This juvenile boa constrictor is displaying a behaviour known as 'star-gazing'.
i. What is your interpretation of this behaviour?
ii. How can this physical sign be employed in formulating a tentative diagnosis and prognosis for recovery?

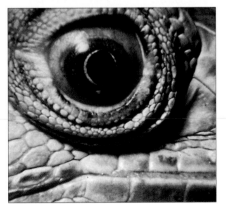

112 The sclerae of this 14-year-old male common green iguana have become progressively brown during the past few months. The lizard's appetite and stools are normal and its vital signs are normal.
i. What is your diagnosis?
ii. What is the significance of the pigmented sclerae?

110 i. Severe icterus.
ii. Liver, gall bladder and/or biliary drainage tract.

111 i. Meningoencephalitis.
ii. 'Star-gazing' is a grave sign because nervous tissue, once damaged, does not regenerate. When the cells of the central nervous system are destroyed, they are not replaced; therefore, recovery is unlikely. Although amoebic, bacterial and mycotic pathogens have been found to be responsible for the non-specific clinical sign of star-gazing, the aetiologic agents which cause meningoencephalitis in snakes most frequently are viruses, especially paramyxovirus, reovirus and lentivirus, although several others also can induce this serious neurologic sign.

112 i. Melanin pigmentation of the sclerae.
ii. Darkening of the sclerae is a normal, age-related phenomenon in older iguanas and, thus, is of no clinical significance.

113 i. What is the condition affecting this snake's integument?
ii. How would you treat this disorder?
iii. What changes in husbandry practices would you recommend that might help prevent this condition?

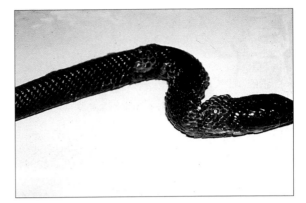

114 i. Identify this blood cell from a spiny-tailed iguana.
ii. What is its function?

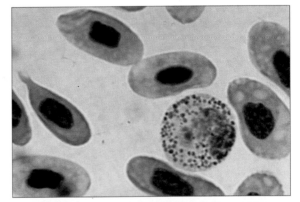

115 These two three-year-old female red-eared slider turtles are being kept under different captive husbandry conditions. The turtle on the right is normal.
i. What is your diagnosis of the turtle on the left?
ii. What poor techniques of captive management might be the cause of this turtle's disorder?
iii. How is this condition treated?

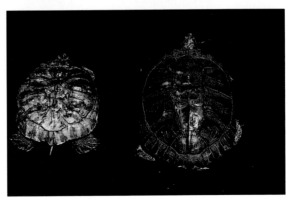

113 i. Vesicular dermatitis ('blister' disease).
ii. Give parenteral bacteriocidal antibiotic therapy, supportive fluid-replacement therapy, and repeated soaking in 0.75% chlorhexidine solution for 30 minutes daily until the skin has healed completely.
iii. Although this is an infectious bacterial disorder, its development usually follows confinement of reptiles under filthy and moist captive conditions. Therefore, cage hygiene is essential.

114 i. Heterophil granulocyte. Note the numerous small brownish granules and slightly pale basophilic cytoplasm.
ii. Heterophils serve as phagocytes, act in response to chemotactic stimulus, and release lytic enzymes.

115 i. Metabolic bone disease.
ii. A diet rich in phosphorus and low in calcium; hypovitaminosis D_3; and lack of exposure to unfiltered sunlight or full-spectrum ultraviolet light can cause metabolic bone disease.
iii. Change to a more natural high-calcium, moderate-phosphorus diet that contains bony tissue, eg, live fish or commercial floating turtle chow, and calcium-rich leafy vegetation and algae. If deemed appropriate, calcium lactate or gluconate can be administered orally or parenterally (1.0–2.5mg/kg daily). Although the bony carapace and plastron will eventually become remineralised when the turtle's diet is improved, the deformities are likely to remain apparent for the life of the turtle.

116 This adult female iguana (**right**) has bilateral lesions over her shoulders.
i. What is your diagnosis of this condition?
ii. What is the significance of these lesions?
iii. As a predictor of future events, what can you forecast to her owner?

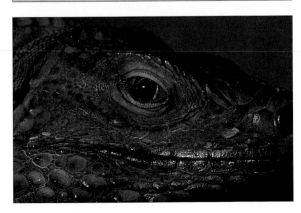

117 Which of the following formed elements of reptilian blood is the granulocyte whose biological activity is functionally analogous to the polymorphonuclear neutrophil in mammals?
i. The basophil.
ii. The eosinophil.
iii. The histiocytic macrophage.
iv. The thrombocyte.
v. The heterophil.

118 This ovum was observed during the microscopic examination of the faeces of an Australian bearded dragon lizard.
i. What is your diagnosis?
ii. What is the treatment?

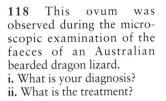

119 The sclerae of this half-grown Caribbean rhinoceros iguana are bright red. The iguana's vision appears to be normal and it is not scratching at its eyes. What is your diagnosis?

116 i. Bite trauma sustained when the iguana was grasped by a male's jaws during copulation.
ii. The iguana is gravid and the eggs are probably fertile.
iii. The coelom will continue to become distended until the clutch of eggs is deposited. Therefore, a suitable incubation area supplied with an appropriate incubation medium should be prepared.

117 v. The heterophil.

118 i. Oxyurid helminth (pinworm) ovum.
ii. Pyrantel pamoate (5mg/kg orally, repeated after two weeks) is effective. Thiabendazole (50mg/kg), febendazole (50mg/kg), mebendazole (20mg/kg) and levamisole (5mg/kg) are equally effective.

119 This species (and several others) of Caribbean iguana normally possesses bright red sclerae. Therefore, no treatment is necessary.

120 A green rat snake has an intracoelomic swelling in the region of the heart. Paracentesis discloses the presence of turbid fluid.
i. What is your tentative diagnosis?
ii. With what two alternative diagnoses might this condition be confused?
iii. How could you determine the exact diagnosis?

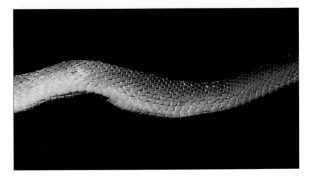

121 The Burmese python (**below, left**) and the rosy boa (**below, right**) display an essentially identical pathological condition.
i. What is your diagnosis?
ii. What is the aetiology of this disorder?
iii. How would you treat this condition?
iv. What is the prognosis for this condition?

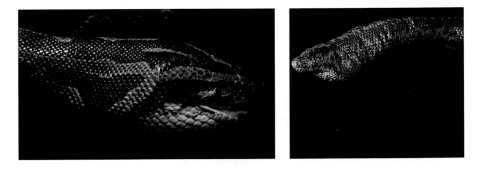

122 When handling reptiles, why is it imperative to support the mass of the body so as not to impose excessive force or traction to the cervical and cephalic parts of the skeleton?

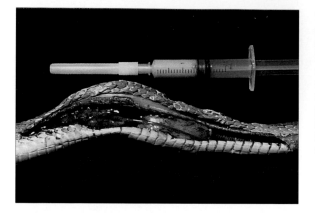

120 i. A fluid pus-filled abscess (left).
ii. Alternative diagnoses include: neoplasia, parasitic and other forms of acquired cyst(s), and gastric hypertrophy secondary to cryptosporidiosis.
iii. Cytology, Gram staining, and microbiological culture of aspirated fluid.

121 i. Intermandibular cellulitis.
ii. The synergistic effects of *Pseudomonas fluorescens* and *Aeromonas hydrophila* infection.
iii. This condition requires aggressive therapy which includes potent bacteriocidal antibiotics, supportive physiological fluid replacement, the provision of additional warmth, and compassionate nursing care. Experimentally, this dual infection has responded well to butirosin sulphate therapy; however, at the date of this book's publication, this drug is not available commercially.
iv. Guarded to unfavourable.

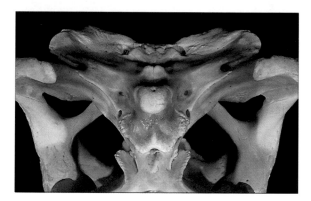

122 Reptiles have a single occipital condyle supporting their skull (left). If too much force is applied to their skull, brainstem and spinal cord, trauma can be induced. Therefore, it is imperative to support a reptile's mass so as not to place undue force on the head and cervical spine when picking up and/or restraining it.

123 This whole-body radiograph is of an adult desert tortoise, which was anorectic, anaemic, and clinically blind.
i. What is your diagnosis?
ii. How would you confirm your diagnosis?
iii. What is your treatment of this disorder?

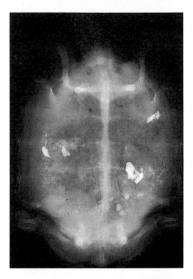

124 The greyish-white, semi-solid urinary excretion of terrestrial reptiles differs markedly from that of most mammals.
i. What is the microcrystalline substance which forms the bulk of the urinary excretory product?
ii. How does this difference affect the manner in which you would treat your reptilian patients?

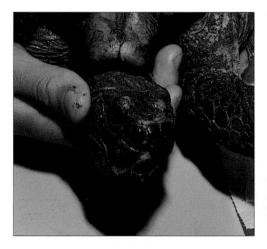

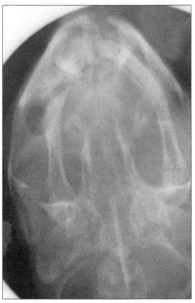

125 The head of a tortoise (above, left) is shown immediately following severe trauma to its mandible, premaxilla, maxilla and nasal bones. The radiograph (right) is of the same tortoise's head.
i. What are the immediate priorities for management?
ii. How would you manage this case for the longer term?
iii. What is the prognosis?

123 i. Multiple metallic objects are present in the alimentary tract. These were found to be chips of lead-based paint that caused lead poisoning.

ii. Chemical determination of the amount of lead in the blood. The plasma contained 211mcg/dl of lead (control tortoise's plasma – 25.7mcg/dl).

iii. Remove the lead fragments from the stomach with an endoscope and long forceps. Administer sodium calciumedetate (35mg/kg daily for two weeks by slow intravenous infusion using a butterfly needle-set placed into the jugular vein).

124 i. Urates (uric acid salts of sodium, ammonium, calcium, and potassium).

ii. Because most terrestrial reptiles are essentially uricotelic and because urate salts are poorly soluble, it is extremely important to maintain hydration and plasma volume when treating sick reptiles so that drug agents do not accumulate to reach toxic concentrations. Many sick reptiles will not drink voluntarily and, thus, should be treated parenterally.

125 i. Maintain a patent airway; if necessary, insert an endotracheal catheter; control haemorrhage; treat any ophthalmic or other soft tissue injuries; look for signs of traumatic or hypovolaemic shock, and treat as necessary.

ii. Once the tortoise is stabilised, anaesthetise it with an oxygen/nitrous oxide/isoflurane mixture; repair the multiple maxillofacial and mandibular fractures by interfragmentary wiring (**below, left**); and stabilise the wires with cold-setting dental acrylic. The tortoise is shown immediately after the endotracheal tube was removed (**below, right**). The dental acrylic was finally removed approximately two years after the fractures were repaired.

iii. Favourable. However, this type of case may require long-term intensive and compassionate care by the owner or keeper. In this case the tortoise had to be handfed and watered for almost two years, demonstrating that with a committed owner, even massively traumatised animals can often be salvaged to recover and thrive afterward.

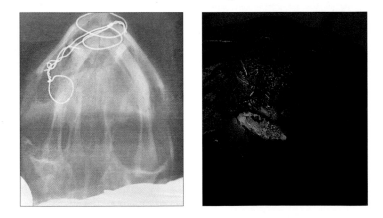

126 The kidneys of a rat snake during necropsy are shown.
i. What is your diagnosis?
ii. What are the two most likely causes for this condition in captive snakes?

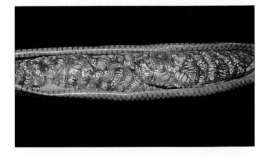

127 i. What is your diagnosis of the condition seen in this juvenile boa constrictor?
ii. How would you treat this condition?
iii. How may it be prevented?

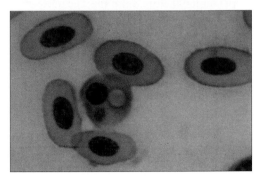

128 This Wright's-stained blood film is from an East African chameleon. One of the cells contains objects in addition to a nucleus.
i. What is your diagnosis?
ii. What is the significance of this condition?

129 In one major respect, amphibian and reptilian blood differs markedly from that of mammals. This is important to know when processing, examining and interpreting a blood specimen from an amphibian or reptile.
i. What is this major difference?
ii. Why is it important to know this when employing an automated instrument used for counting blood cells?

126 i. Urate deposition.
ii. (1) Dehydration-induced visceral gout; (2) iatrogenic aminoglycoside-induced nephrosis and visceral gout, leading to hyperuricaemia and urate accumulation.

127 i. Dysecdysis.
ii. The boa should be soaked for at least 30 minutes in mildly tepid water, then 'sandwiched' between layers of moistened towelling so that the now-moisturised epidermis can be loosened and removed as the boa crawls through the cloth. If necessary, a few drops of hard-contact lens-wetting solution can be placed on the retained tertiary spectacles to enhance their moisturisation.
iii. Furnish the boa's cage with a water container sufficiently large to permit it to bathe, and one or more large rocks or logs upon which it can rub its chin to initiate the moulting process.

128 i. Chameleon erythrocyte virus infection. This is an iridovirus.
ii. Although many chameleons may exhibit these inclusions, which are viral assemblages, most do not appear to be affected. However, if a chameleon is sufficiently stressed or infected with other pathogens, this agent may contribute to illness.

129 i. The formed cellular constituents of amphibian and reptilian blood retain their nuclei during their maturation. The nuclei of erythrocytes and thrombocytes are elongated and oval, and, sometimes, have scalloped shapes; the nuclei of lymphocytes and azurophils are usually round; the nuclei of monocytes are often indented and horseshoe-shaped; and the nuclei of heterophilic, basophilic and eosinophilic granulocytes may be single and smooth-edged, or multi-lobed.
ii. Because all of the blood cells are nucleated, automated cell counters will yield erroneous results. To obviate this problem, special stain-containing diluents have been developed to be used when counting nucleated blood cells in a haemocytometer.

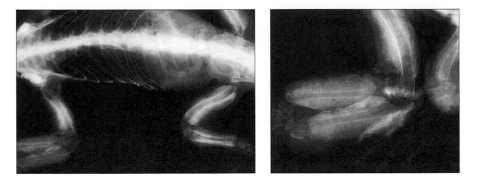

130 An adult male common green iguana had become progressively reluctant to bear weight on its limbs. The iguana could walk, but only with great difficulty. Physical examination revealed that all four limbs were swollen and very tender to even the most gentle digital palpation. Bilateral slightly raised longitudinal ridges were seen on the rib cage, particularly when the iguana took in a deep breath. The diet was nutritious consisting of leafy vegetables and small amounts of canned cat food and primate biscuits. The iguana was permitted to roam the owners' home and had learned to use the clay-based litter-filled trays provided for the household cats. The results of haematology and clinical chemistry investigations are given. The radiographs show the limbs (**above, left**) and the distal left humerus, radius and ulna (**above, right**).

Haematology

Test	Results	One month later	Normal value(s)
WBC	16.3 x 10³/mm³	8.2 x 10³/mm³	12–22.5 x 10³/mm³
PCV	20%	35%	16–30%
Haemoglobin	nd	nd	4.8–11.9
NucRBC/100	0	nd	N/A
Metamyelos	4/10³µl	0/10³µl	N/A
Bands	4/10³µl	0/10³µl	N/A
Azurophils	61/10³µl	28/10³µl	0–20
Lymphocytes	31/10³µl	71/10³µl	21–91
Monocytes	0	0	0–10
Eosinophils	0	0	0–3
Basophils	0	0	0–3
Thrombocytes	Adequate	Adequate	

Clinical chemistry

Test	Results	Ten days later	Normal value(s)
Serum SGOT(AST)	213 µl	253µ/l	200–300
Glucose	133 mg/dl	nd mg/dl	<155
Phosphorus	nd mg/dl	nd mg/dl	5.8–6.7
Calcium	9.7 mg/dl	nd mg/dl	11.6–13.8
Total protein	4.0 mg/dl	2.8 mg/dl	4.5
Uric acid	8.1 mg/dl	6.8 mg/dl	<5.0

i. What is your diagnosis?
ii. What is the underlying pathogenesis of this condition?
iii. What is the prognosis for this disorder?

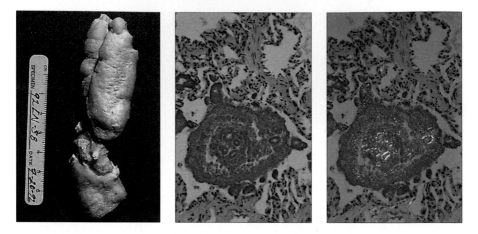

130 i. Hypertrophic pulmonary osteoarthropathy (HPOA). An osteologic specimen of one forelimb is shown (**above, left**). The paired photomicrographs (**above, centre** and **above, right**) are of pulmonary tissue under plain and cross-polarised illumination respectively. Note the refractile mineral fibres in the third figure.

ii. The following histopathological lesions were observed: massive pulmonary silicosis and fibrosis; severe hepatic fibrosis; interstitial nephritis and fibrosis; non-suppurative thyroiditis; and medial arteriosclerosis. Which one or which combination of these significant pathological conditions induced the severe hypertrophic osteoarthropathy in this lizard is conjectural, because almost any of the lesions could have been responsible. However, the severity of the pulmonary and hepatic pathologies make the lung and the liver likely candidates. When this case was investigated epidemiologically, the origin of the pulmonary silicosis was revealed to be a high-silica content commercial cat litter which, on microscopic comparison with the microcrystalline mineral found in the lungs of this iguana, was shown to be identical.

To summarise, this interesting case could have been diagnosed most effectively by its characteristic radiographic abnormalities. The haematological and clinical chemistry investigations did not contribute information that was organ-specific with respect to the induction of the severe osseous pathology. In retrospect, perhaps blood gas studies might have demonstrated pulmonary dysfunction and systemic hypoxaemia. Similarly, serum alkaline and acid phosphatase determinations might have disclosed gross alterations due to bone matrix turnover. Had a liver biopsy been performed, it would have revealed massive hepatic fibrosis, but no clue to the pulmonary silicosis would have been provided without a lung biopsy (which is not a procedure routinely performed in reptiles). If nothing else, this case demonstrates some of the limitations of haematology and clinical chemistry investigations. It does, however, confirm the enormous value of obtaining a thorough history and conducting a careful physical examination.

iii. Guarded to poor unless the cause can be elucidated and corrected.

131 This is a lesion in the eye of a turtle (**right**).
i. What is your diagnosis?
ii. How would you treat this lesion?

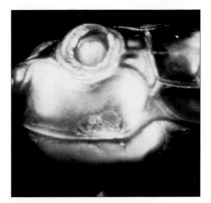

132 The colourful pigmentation of some reptiles' skin (which may be black, brown, red, yellow, green, white, or combinations of any of these hues) is due to a specific cell type from which benign and malignant tumours occasionally arise. What is this cell type?

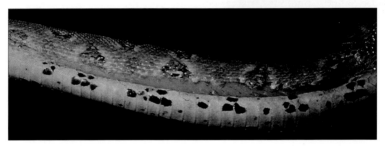

133 This juvenile boa constrictor (**above**) has been fed live rats that have been kept without food for 6–8 hours (the interval between purchase and when the rodents were offered to the snake). While swallowing one of these rats, the skin of the lateral area of the snake's neck suddenly ruptured.
i. What is your diagnosis of this condition?
ii. Why is it important to know that the prey of this snake have not been fed for several hours?
iii. How would you treat this traumatic skin rupture?
iv. What measures should be taken to avoid a repetition of this disorder?

134 This desert tortoise has a rostral protruberance which has been growing slowly for several years.
i. What is your diagnosis?
ii. How would you treat this condition?

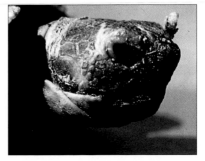

131 i. Hypopyon.
ii. Parenteral therapy with a bacteriocidal broad-spectrum antibiotic, and topical instillation of an ophthalmic ointment that contains both a compatible antibiotic and a corticosteroid.

132 Chromatophores. Those that contain black or brown pigment are called melanophores; red pigment cells are called erythrophores; those that contain yellow pigment granules are called xanthophores; and those which impart a white or silvery hue are called iridophores. Combinations of two or more chromatophore types yield shades of tan, orange, pink, green, etc.

133 i. Spontaneous skin rupture, possibly due to hypovitaminosis C.
ii. Under natural conditions, snakes consume prey that have been eating normally; thus, when they consume their prey, the snakes also benefit from the contents of their prey's alimentary system. Although most snakes synthesise vitamin C in varying amounts, occasionally, these amounts are insufficient to meet a particular snake's metabolic requirements for this vitamin. In rodents, vitamin C synthesis occurs in the gut; so, if prey rodents have not eaten prior to being fed to snakes, their bodies lack the vital vitamin C-containing ingesta and faeces.
iii. The traumatic laceration must be debrided and sutured, and the snake must be given vitamin C parenterally for several days.
iv. If freshly-killed rodents are used as prey, they should be fed a meal prior to being offered to a snake. Alternatively, if frozen and then thawed rodents are used, an appropriate amount of vitamin C in the form of sodium ascorbate can be injected into the rodent carcase, or a portion of a vitamin C tablet can be inserted into the rodent carcase so that it will be absorbed when the snake swallows and digests the meal.

134 i. Cutaneous horn.
ii. Because of their potential to promote the formation of malignant cutaneous neoplasms, these excrescent lesions should be excised along with a cuff of normal full-thickness integument.

135 This is a coeliotomy in an adult female desert tortoise.
i. What is the dark structure being pointed at with the scalpel?
ii. Is this structure vital to the tortoise?

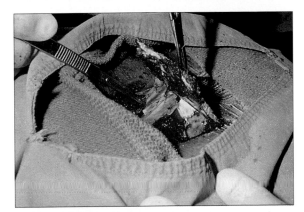

136 This juvenile monitor lizard has a **unilateral** blepharospasm. The lizard resists inspection and/or treatment for this condition. How would you manage this case?

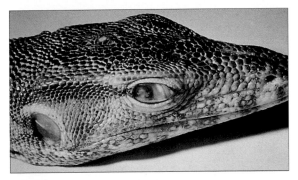

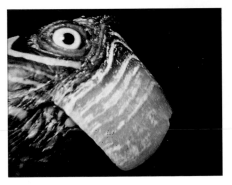

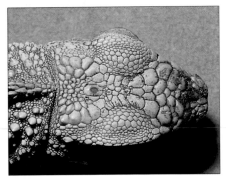

137 This chelonian (**above**) has a condition affecting its maxillary mouthpart.
i. What is your diagnosis?
ii. How would you treat it?
iii. What measures should be taken to prevent this problem?

138 In some lizards and the tuatara, the paired lateral eyes are augmented by another sense organ (**above**).
i. What is this organ?
ii. What is the function of this structure?

135 i. One of the paired ventral abdominal veins.
ii. No. If absolutely necessary, both veins can be double-ligated and divided without causing harm to the patient. They should, however, be preserved if possible.

136 The conjunctival sac and surrounding ocular and periocular tissues can be thoroughly examined and evaluated only under anaesthesia. Once the lizard is anaesthetised, its eyelids are opened and the conjunctival sac is inspected. The piece of inspissated exudate found wedged beneath the lower eyelid, which is preventing the lid from being lowered, should be flushed from its site with a stream of sterile saline. Once the dried exudate is removed, an ophthalmic antibiotic ointment can be instilled into the conjunctival sac. The owner should be instructed to repeat this treatment three times daily for one week.

137 i. Malocclusion.
ii. The redundant horny maxillary tissue must be trimmed so that the normal shearing action of the two jaws is restored. Using a power-driven saw, shorten the excessive tomia; then create a relatively sharp edge by sanding the freshly cut tomia with a shaft-mounted sanding drum or disc.
iii. Feed a more natural diet that contains hard items, eg, shelled molluscs. Alternatively, feed the tortoise on an abrasive surface, eg, concrete, so that each time it eats, it abrades its mouth parts slightly; or trim its mouth parts periodically with an emery board or medium-grit abrasive paper.

138 i. The parietal eye.
ii. The parietal eye detects shadows and, thus, perceives the potential threat of predators. It also serves as a dosimeter of light and, as such, helps regulate the diurnal basking activities of reptiles that possess these accessory light-sensitive organs.

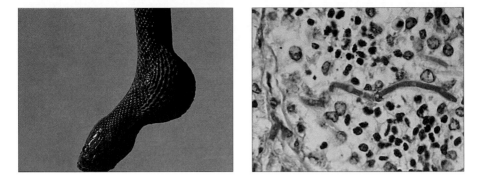

139 This corn snake developed a soft, fluctuant mass beneath its integument (**above, left**). A biopsy specimen stained with haematoxylin and eosin revealed the structures illustrated (**above, right**).
i. What is your diagnosis?
ii. What is your treatment?

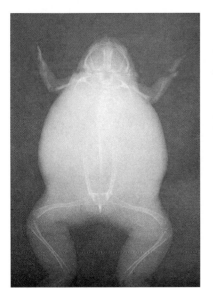

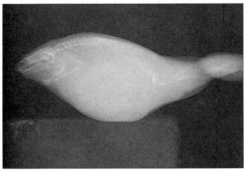

140 The dorsoventral and left lateral projection radiographs of a mature African clawed frog that displayed marked coelomic distension are shown.
i. What is your diagnosis?
ii. How would you treat this frog?

141 As a group, reptiles have highly varied diets and specialised nutritional requirements. What essential vitamins are not synthesised by healthy reptiles and therefore must be ingested either as a precursor molecule or as the preformed product?

139 i. Mycetoma; fungal granuloma
ii. After the biopsy results are obtained, the snake should be re-anaesthetised and the mass and as much normal tissue immediately surrounding it should be excised. Flush the cavity remaining at the site of the mass several times with dilute povidone iodine solution, and install a drain before closing the surgical defect. Flush dilute povidone iodine solution into the site through the drain twice daily for five to seven days. In this corn snake, the lesion healed *per primum* after 12 days and did not recur.

Note the large unbranched, septate mycelium and the mixed, mostly mononuclear, leucocytic inflammatory cells that characterise this granulomatous lesion.

140 i. Ascites and hydrops.
ii. Furosemide (frusemide) by injection (5mg/kg daily in two divided doses). Although the frog improved slightly, euthanasia was carried out at the owner's request. Necropsy disclosed bilateral renal adenocarcinoma.

141 Vitamins A and K.

142 These elongated organisms were found during a microscopic examination of faeces from a tegu lizard. The specimen is suspended in potassium dichromate solution.
i. What is your diagnosis?
ii. How would you treat this lizard for this condition?
iii. What instructions should you give to the lizard's owner?

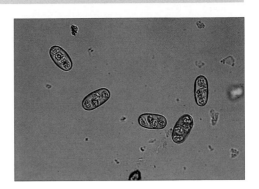

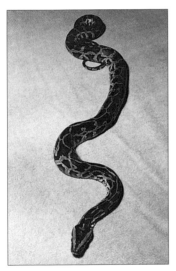

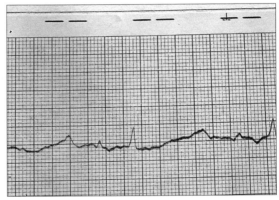

143 A juvenile Burmese python (above, left) was presented for examination because it developed a steadily enlarging heart that could be seen easily when it was at rest. An ECG tracing (above, right) was obtained.
i. What major abnormality is evident in the ECG of this snake?
ii. What is one possible cardiac abnormality that is consistent with this ECG?

144 Female reptiles occasionally experience difficulty in depositing their shelled eggs or fetuses. This condition is termed dystocia. What are some of the reasons for this disorder?

142 i. *Eimeria* sp.

ii. Trimethoprim-sulphamethoxyzole or trimethoprim-sulphadiazine orally (10–20mg/kg daily for one week); or sulphaquinoxyline, sulphamethazine, sulphamerazine, or sulphadimethoxine (60–90mg/kg on the first day, followed by 45mg/kg for the next six days).

iii. All faeces must be removed promptly so that the lizard does not become reinfected by any oocysts that escaped eradication during the first treatment.

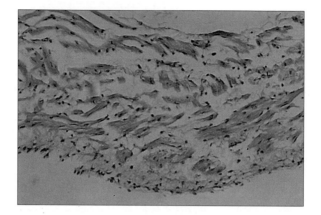

143 i. First-degree heart block.

ii. Any of several conditions can result in conduction disturbances. Usually, the origin of the disturbance is in the atrium. In this instance, the python had a developmental defect consisting of myocardial hypoplasia affecting both of the atria and the single ventricle (**above**). Other aetiologies for this form of heart block are: some chemical and plant intoxications, hypoxia, hypoglycaemia, potassium depletion, thyrotoxicosis, atrial ectopic beats, atrial fibrillation, myocardial ischaemia, congestive heart failure, and several miscellaneous endogenous cardiomyopathies.

144 • Oviductal disease such as infection, adhesions or stenosis.
  • Necrotic eggs of embryos (or fetuses).
  • Fractured eggshells.
  • Abnormally sized or shaped shelled ova, embryos or fetuses.
  • Abnormally narrowed pelvic canal (in all reptiles except snakes and legless lizards).
  • Hypocalcaemia.
  • Lack of a suitable site in which to deposit eggs.
  • Disturbance-induced stress.

145 i. Identify this basophilic cell.
ii. What clinical conditions
should be suspected when
many of these cells are
found in a reptile's blood?

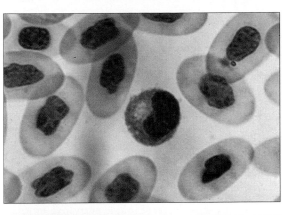

146 These two adult
Galapagos tortoises (**right**)
were fed a diet of mixed
vegetables, with a prepon-
derance of cabbage, for over
one year. All the tortoises
within the collection who
were fed the same diet display similar lesions.
i. What is your diagnosis?
ii. What causes this con-
dition?
iii. What is the treatment for
this disorder?
iv. What measures can be
taken to prevent it?

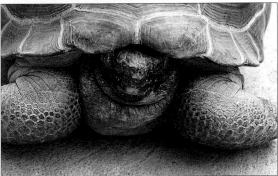

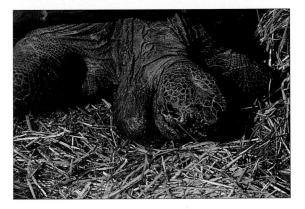

145 i. Plasmacyte.

ii. An immunogenic response to an antigenic challenge – for example, chronic infection – would cause an increase in plasmacytes in the blood. Also, a monoclonal plasmacytic neoplasm should be considered. Serum electrophoresis would help elucidate plasmacytic myeloproliferation by revealing an abnormal globulin fraction distribution.

146 i. Hypothyroidism leading to the formation of fibrous goitres.

ii. In this instance, the feeding of a diet consisting mostly of cabbage (which contains goitrogens) induces diminished function of the thyroid gland and its synthesis and secretion of thyroxin. This is a condition common to herbivorous reptiles that have evolved in volcanic island habitats in which halogen- (iodine, chlorine, fluorine and bromine) sequestrating plants predominate over those that do not concentrate halogens in their tissues.

iii. Administer a source of iodine every five to seven days, eg, sodium- or potassium iodide solution (0.25–0.50mg/kg i/v or orally) or Lugol's solution (0.5–2.0mg/kg orally).

iv. Supplement the diet with kelp tablets; the dosage of this form of iodine is not critical because kelp is essentially non-toxic when used as a dietary supplement for giant tortoises. Depending upon their iodine content, a 150–200kg tortoise could be given three to six tablets weekly.

147 This parasitic organism was extracted from the subcutis of an Asian snake.
i. What is it?
ii. What is your treatment for this condition?
iii. What is the life cycle of this parasite?

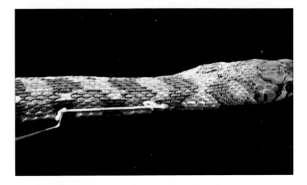

148 This Pacific pond turtle has a particularly striking lesion involving its left forelimb.
i. What is your diagnosis?
ii. What is the cause of this lesion?
iii. What is the significance of this lesion?
iv. What advice should you offer to the owner?

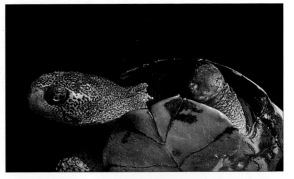

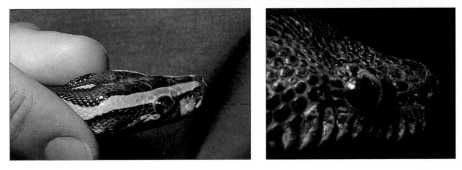

149 The juvenile royal python (**above, left**) and the Malagasy tree boa (**above, right**) have essentially identical ophthalmic lesions.
i. What is your diagnosis?
ii. How would you treat these lesions?

147 i. A plerocercoid (larval form) of *Spirometra* sp.

ii. Remove the immature stages of the cestode from their subcuticular sites of encystment. Administer praziquantel (5–8mg/kg i/m, repeated after two weeks). Feed only live prey items proven to be free of parasitism or, if that is not possible, feed only thawed frozen prey that has been held at a subfreezing temperature for a minimum of 30 days.

iii. The ova shed in the faeces are ingested by copepods; these are ingested by fish or amphibian larvae which are then ingested by reptiles. The infected reptile is ingested by a mammal in which the adult tapeworms develop to sexual maturity.

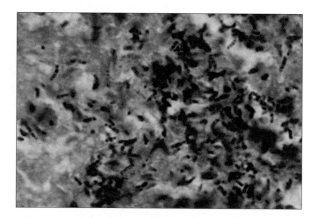

148 i. Mycobacteriosis; lepromatous leprosy.

ii. *Mycobacterium* spp. Note the myriad number of acid-fast bacilli (**above**).

iii. Several species of acid-fast microorganisms have been associated with similar lesions in semi-aquatic chelonians. Some, if not most, of these microorganisms are pathogenic for humans. Therefore, this turtle is a public health hazard.

iv. Euthanasia of all suspected Mycobacteria-infected chelonians.

149 i. Bullous spectaculopathy. Fluid has accumulated behind and is distending the affected tertiary spectacles in these snakes.

ii. Sometimes, these lesions are self limiting. In cases where the condition remains static or becomes worse, the ballooned spectacle can be excised circumferentially where it joins the integument at the rim of the orbit. Treat the now-exposed cornea topically with a corticosteroid/antibiotic ophthalmic ointment until healing is completed. Usually, a new spectacle will form prior to the next moult.

150 i. What is the parasite in this histopathological photomicrograph? Hint: note that it lacks a coelom and a digestive tract.
ii. What would your treatment be for this parasite?

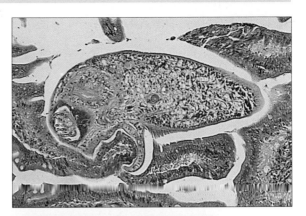

151 This adult tree frog has a condition affecting its premaxilla and palate.
i. What is your diagnosis?
ii. How would you treat the frog for this condition?
iii. What is the prognosis?

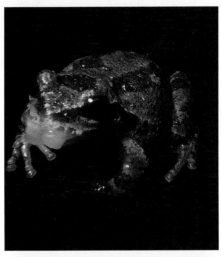

152 What are the paired lobed structures in the caudal third of the coelomic cavity of this snake's cadaver?

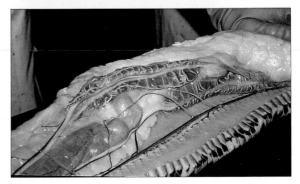

150 i. An acanthocephalan helminth. Note the refractile thorn-like hooks on its rostral end.
ii. Ivermectin (200mcg/kg i/m or orally, repeated after two weeks).

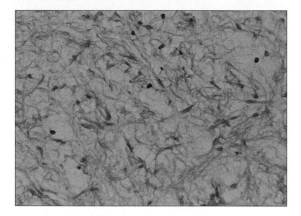

151 i. The frog has a myxoma, a proliferative neoplastic lesion that occurs frequently in tree frogs.
ii. Because these tumours often make it difficult for affected frogs to catch and consume their insect prey, this frog should be anaesthetised and the mass excised.
iii. Favourable. Although these benign myxomatous tumours often recur after subtotal excision, their progression is slow and, since the normal life-span of these tree frogs is usually short, most frogs complete a relatively normal life after the myxomata have been removed.

The histological section of the tumour (**above**) illustrates the characteristic multipolar cells imbedded in a poorly staining finely fibrillar mucoid ground substance - (H & E stain, x76 original magnification).

152 Kidneys.

153 This is an ophthalmic lesion in a desert tortoise. The photograph was taken in the early spring shortly after the chelonian emerged from hibernation.
i. What is your diagnosis?
ii. How would you treat this condition?
iii. What is the prognosis?

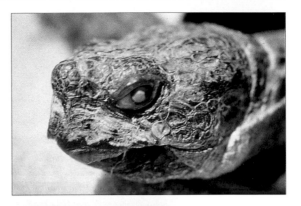

154 How would you manage the mid-shaft femoral fracture illustrated in this radiograph of a mature iguana?

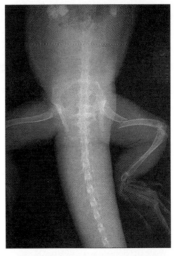

155 This parasitic ovum was found in the faeces of a Timor monitor lizard.
i. What kind of parasite is it?
ii. What is your treatment to eradicate this organism?
iii. What kind of intermediate host does this parasite employ during its development?

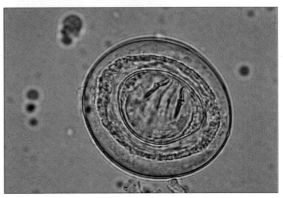

153 i. Post-hibernation corneal coagulative plaques.

ii. These lesions respond very well to topical instillation of a proteolytic ophthalmic ointment two to three times daily. Usually, these corneal lesions are completely healed after seven days treatment.

iii. Favourable. However, some chelonians sustain concomitant neurologic damage after being exposed to severely low temperatures during hibernation. Although their corneal lesions may heal, they may remain blind due to nerve damage.

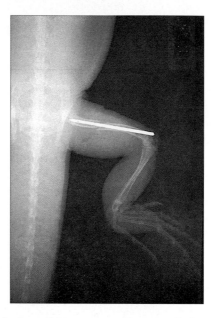

154 Intramedullary pinning with an appropriate-size Steinmann pin (**above**). Note that this iguana's leg was broken as a result of accidental trauma and not metabolic bone disease. The cortical bone is well mineralised and, thus, could support an intramedullary pin for internal support.

155 i. A cestode (tapeworm) ovum.

ii. Praziquantel (8mg/kg orally, repeated after two weeks).

iii. Likely intermediate hosts include arthropods and rodents.

156 This boa constrictor is one of a group being kept in a breeding colony. All of the snakes in this collection were behaving abnormally. When placed upon their backs, most remained stationary for a prolonged period. Many appeared to be clinically blind. Some had various respiratory and oral infections before developing bizarre behaviour patterns. The onset of these signs was sudden and followed the introduction of an adult male boa that was on breeding loan.

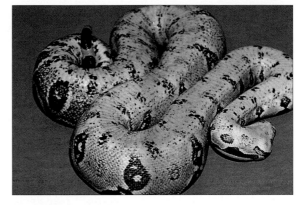

i. What is your diagnosis?
ii What is the prognosis?
iii What control measure(s) should be instituted to prevent this disorder?

157 This Wright's-stained blood film (**centre, right**) is from a mature female Russell's viper that has rapidly declined in health over a period of six weeks. What is your interpretation of the blood film?

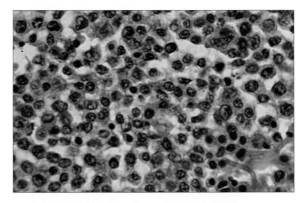

158 i. What does the radiograph (**right**) of the hindlimbs and thoracolumbar vertebrae of this young adult iguana reveal?.
ii. How would you treat this condition?

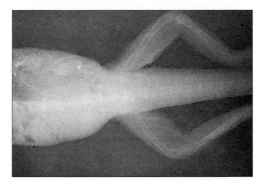

156 i. Encephalitis. The aetiology was probably infectious. Any of the following four viruses could have been the causative agent: lentivirus, reovirus, paramyxovirus or herpesvirus.
ii. Guarded to grave.
iii. All affected snakes should be euthanised and necropsied. If possible, samples should be collected for virologic and electron microscopic investigations. All cages and their furnishings must be thoroughly disinfected to kill any residual infective agents. No snakes, even those that are not displaying signs of disease, should be removed from the premises, and no newly acquired snakes or snakes borrowed on breeding loan should be added to the colony without completing a rigorous quarantine period during which a thorough screening for pathogens is accomplished.

157 Myelogenous leukaemia. Note the numerous atypical and anaplastic leukocytes, some of which contain nuclei in mitosis. Chemotherapy might have been considered if this patient had been a mammal or even a non-venomous snake; however, because she was a long-term captive, highly venomous snake, she was euthanised and subjected to complete pathological investigation.

158 i. 'Folding'-type fracture of the popliteal region of the left distal femur and a generalised osteopenia involving the long bone cortices.
ii. This type of fracture usually heals without external splintage. The diet should be improved so that the calcium content is richer in relation to phosphorus. The iguana should receive periodic exposure to unfiltered sunlight or artificial full-spectrum ultraviolet illumination or, alternatively, its diet should be supplemented with vitamin D_3.

159 This diamondback terrapin has a disorder involving its mouth parts.
i. What is your diagnosis?
ii. How would you treat this condition?
iii. What measures can be taken to prevent this condition from recurring?

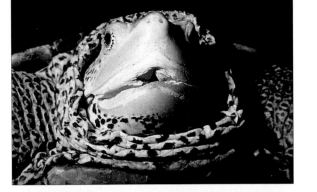

160 This Argentine horned frog had been apparently healthy before being found one morning as illustrated .
i. What is your diagnosis of this condition?
ii. What is the most expedient method for correcting this condition?
iii. How can this particular frog be treated to prevent this disorder from recurring?

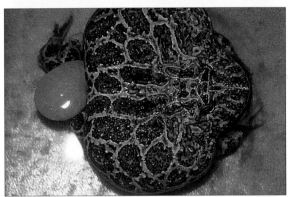

161 i. What condition is evident in the caudal region of this immature boa constrictor?
ii. What is a likely aetiology for this condition?
iii. How would you treat it?

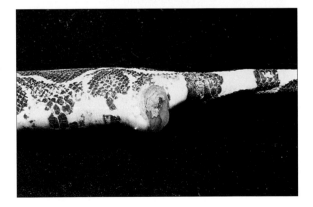

159 i. Malocclusion due to the accumulation of keratinous debris.

ii. With only manual restraint being necessary, hold the terrapin's mouth open and, using a small dental instrument, remove the accumulated debris. These deposits lift away easily from the subjacent normal oral tissues.

iii. In their natural habitat, the diet of these terrapins consists mainly of small marine molluscs, such as periwinkles and other snail-like shelled invertebrates. When these molluscs are consumed, their hard shells abrade the terrapins' oral tissues, thus keeping them free of excessive keratin debris. The diet fed to captive chelonians should include food items that are mildly abrasive – small periwinkle-type marine snails and/or dry commercial turtle or trout chow are suitable for this purpose.

160 i. Eversion and prolapse of the urinary bladder.

ii. The prolapsed tissue should be gently cleansed with a non-cytotoxic antiseptic solution, eg, 0.75% chlorhexidine. The contents of the urinary bladder should be aspirated, and the prolapse can be reduced by using a smooth instrument or cotton-tipped applicator.

iii. Carry out a percutaneous cystopexy by inserting a small instrument or cotton-tipped applicator into the urinary bladder and, using it as a guide, place two to three full thickness through-and-through stapling sutures to fix the bladder wall to the inner surface of the adjacent belly wall.

161 i. Prolapse of the cloacal membrane.

ii. Any irritation that would encourage the boa to strain might induce such a prolapse, eg, constipation or obstipation, intestinal parasitism, cloacitis and foreign bodies that adhere to the exposed mucous membranes at the time of defaecation.

iii. Cleanse the exposed moist surfaces with an appropriate non-cytotoxic antiseptic; lubricate the mucosa; replace the cloacal membrane using a cotton-tipped applicator or similar device as an obturator; and, while the obturator is still in place, insert a purse-string suture circumferentially around the cloacal vent, making certain that it is only sufficiently tight to prevent reprolapse, but not so tight as to impede the passage of faeces and urinary wastes; leave the purse-string suture in place for 10 to 14 days. If prolapse recurs, perform a percutaneous proctopexy, as described in Answer **160**, above.

162 This ovum was found during the microscopic examination of faeces from a tegu lizard.
i. What is this parasite?
ii. What is your treatment for this parasite?

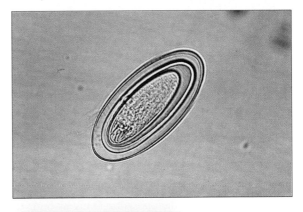

163 i. How would you interpret the radiograph of this mangrove monitor lizard?
ii. What is the possible cause of this condition?
iii. How would you treat this lizard?
iv. What can be done to avoid this condition?

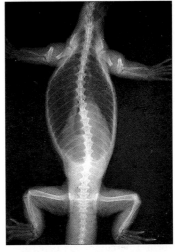

164 This round parasite was found in the faeces of a king snake that was apparently well, but had not eaten for several months.
i. What is this parasite?
ii. How would you treat the snake for this parasite?

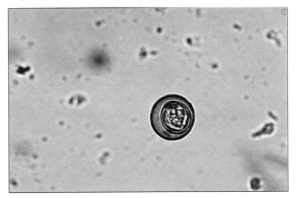

162 i. An acanthocephalan helminth. Note the triple-walled ovum and the hooklets on the rostrum of the embryo.

ii. Ivermectin (200mcg/kg i/m or orally, repeated after two weeks). The faeces should be removed as soon as possible from the cage to avoid reinfestation.

163 i. Bilateral mid-shaft humeral fractures.

ii. Because the skeleton displays adequate mineralisation, it is likely that these bilateral fractures resulted from trauma rather than from poor nutrition. In this case the lizard was physically restrained by having its forelimbs' carpal joints held firmly and brought together so that they were rotated over its back. This restraint technique placed undue force on the humeri, thereby fracturing both of them.

iii. The fractures were immobilised and fixed in end-to-end apposition with human finger-size bone plates and bone screws.

iv. Apply restraint to the upper forelimbs without rotation up and over the cervical and shoulder area. By holding the lizard in this manner, it cannot struggle and injure itself – or its handler.

164 i. *Isospora*.

ii. Trimethoprim-sulphadiazine or trimethoprim-sulphamethoxazole (10–20mg/kg daily for two weeks), or any of several other coccidiostats containing sulpha drugs. Nitrofurans, for example, are equally effective.

165 This adult male Jackson's chameleon has multiple, raised, nodular lesions on its integument.
i. What is your tentative diagnosis?
ii. What tests would you carry out to confirm your diagnosis?
iii. How would you treat it?

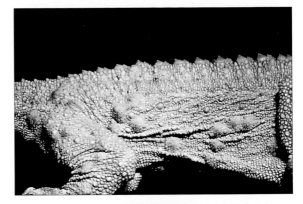

166 i. What is the ophthalmic condition affecting the right eye of this African leopard tortoise?
ii. What is the significance of this condition?

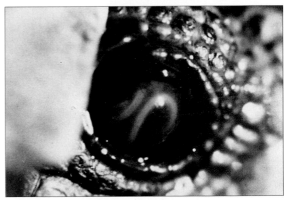

167 i. What is the acute lesion illustrated in this half-grown soft-shelled turtle (a mostly aquatic species)?
ii. What are possible aetiologies for this condition?
iii. How should it be treated?

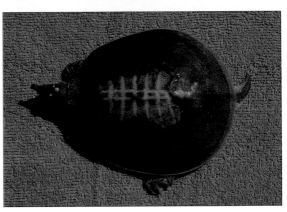

165 i. Mycotic dermatitis.
ii. Excisional biopsy of a typical integumentary lesion – half submitted for histopathology and half submitted for bacteriological and mycological culture and sensitivity testing. In this instance the aetiologic pathogen was *Aspergillus* sp.
iii. Ketoconazole orally (10–30mg/kg daily) and ketoconazole cream topically until the skin lesions are healed. Although Jackson's chameleons require a relatively high environmental humidity, their cages must be kept scrupulously clean in order to prevent an unhealthy habitat.

166 i. There is a helminth within the anterior chamber. This wild-caught African tortoise was infested with filarid worms, one of which had migrated into the eye as a microfilarid and developed to adulthood in this site.
ii. The tortoise can be treated for filariasis, but the eye is permanently damaged.

167 i. Acute necrotising dermatitis.
ii. (1) Thermal injury from an overhead heating device; (2) severe acute or subacute dermatitis.
iii. The denuded tissue should be covered with either an antiseptic waterproof liquid plastic dressing or an antibiotic ointment. In this instance, because this species of turtle is mostly aquatic, the waterproof liquid plastic dressing would be more appropriate.

168 This photomicrograph is of stained iguana blood.
i. What is the small pale-staining cell in the middle of the image?
ii. What is its function?

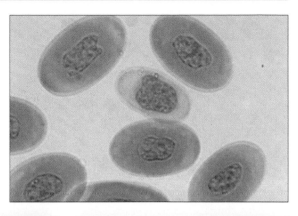

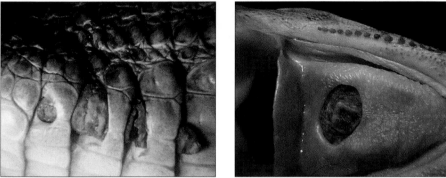

169 A juvenile spectacled caiman is examined and several skin lesions consisting of focal necrosis (**above, left**) are evaluated. Once the necrotic tissue covering each site is removed, the underlying bed of subcuticular tissue appears normal. When the caiman's rostrum is touched, it opens its mouth and reveals a circular necrotic lesion located at the base of its tongue (**above, right**). During digital palpation, the tail feels unusually firm. The diet consists entirely of thawed, frozen herring.
i. What is your diagnosis?
ii. What is the prognosis?
iii. How can this condition be prevented?

170 This ovum was found in the faeces of a blood python.
i. Identify this egg.
ii. How would you treat this snake?

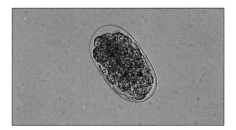

168 i. A thrombocyte.
ii. Thrombocytes are intimately associated with blood clotting. They are also capable of phagocytosis and are pluripotential (able to transform into erythrocytes).

169 i. Steatitis caused by hypovitaminosis E.
ii. The prognosis is guarded because vital visceral tissues and organs may be severely affected. Because of the nature of the granulomatous inflammation that accompanies this disorder, substantial tissue damage and, therefore, dysfunction may occur.
iii. By feeding only fresh foods that do not contain large amounts of saturated fats.

170 i. *Ophiostrongylus* spp.
ii. Ivermectin (200mcg/kg i/m or orally, repeated after two weeks); or pyrantel pamoate (5mg/kg orally, repeated after two weeks); or febendazole (50–100mg/kg orally, repeated after two weeks).

171 A female amelanistic (partial albino) California king snake that has been on public display for 10 years is presented with a firm mass at the ventrolateral aspect of the body wall adjacent to where the ventral belly scutes join the lateral scales. What tests or procedures would you employ to arrive at a diagnosis?

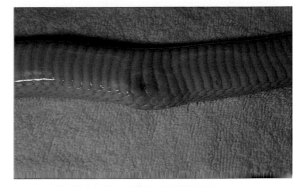

172 This dorsoventral radiograph is of the head of a python.
i. What is your interpretation of this radiograph?
ii. How would you confirm your diagnosis?
iii. How would you treat this python?

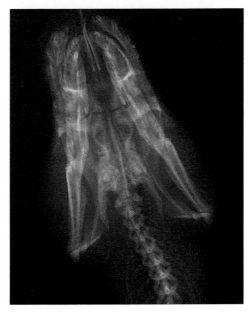

173 i. Identify this cell from a desert tortoise.
ii. What is its biological function?

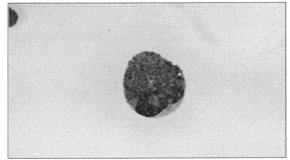

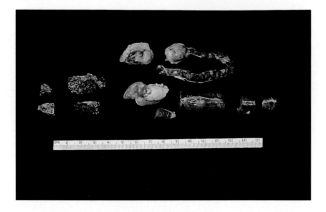

171 Fine-needle percutaneous or open excisional biopsy, histopathology, and micro-biological culture and sensitivity testing. In this instance, an open biopsy was also performed. It was immediately apparent that this mass had extended through the subjacent body wall and into the coelomic cavity. Euthanasia was carried out. Necropsy revealed that most of the major visceral organs (including the liver, pancreas, spleen and both kidneys) had been partially replaced by homogeneous masses of soft white creamy tissue; histopathology revealed the masses to be histiocytic granulomata (**above**).

172 i. Periodontal mandibular osteomyelitis involving several dental alveoli in the left mandibular ramus.
ii. Fine-needle aspiration biopsy of the suspected site of infection; cytological and/or histopathological examination; microbiological culture and antibiotic sensitivity testing.
iii. Surgically debride and lavage the site with 0.75% chlorhexidine solution. Commence parenteral broad-spectrum bacteriostatic antibiotic and fluid-replacement therapy.

173 i. Eosinophil. Note the highly eosinophilic spherical granules and the eccentric non-lobed nucleus.
ii. Eosinophils are attracted by foreign proteinaceous materials and objects, eg, parasites and other immunogens that participate in the stimulation of IgE. When these cells degranulate, they release IgE and antihistaminic substances into the surrounding tissue sites to which they are attracted.

174 These two ova were found during the examination of the faeces from a Gila monster lizard.
i. From what parasite is the thick-shelled round ovum?
ii. From what parasite is the thin-shelled elongated ovum?
iii. What is your treatment to eradicate these parasites?

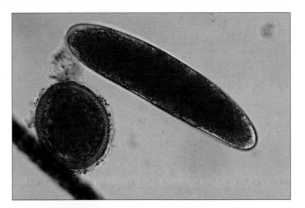

175 An immature common snapping turtle is presented for routine physical examination because it has not been growing. A whole-body radiograph is made.
i. What is your diagnosis?
ii. How would you treat this condition?
iii. What is the aetiology of this disorder?
iv. What long-term measures should be taken?

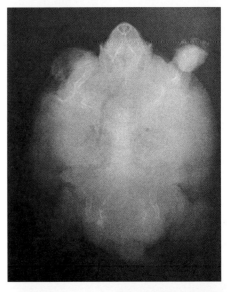

176 This juvenile royal (ball) python is healthy, but one significant lesion can be seen in this view.
i. What is your diagnosis?
ii. Is this condition significant with respect to viability or longevity?
iii. What specific advice would you give to this snake's owner?

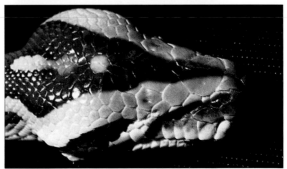

174 i. An ascarid nematode.
ii. A pinworm.
iii. Pyrantel pamoate (5mg/kg, repeated after two weeks); or fenbendazole (50–100mg/kg, repeated after two weeks); or ivermectin (200mcg/kg i/m or orally, repeated after two weeks). To avoid direct reinfestation, the faeces should be removed as soon as possible from the cage.

175 i. Severe osteopenia and osteomalacia; metabolic bone disease; secondary nutritional hyperparathyroidism.
ii. Administer vitamin D_3 orally and 10% calcium gluconate parenterally. Caution: because snapping turtles can be dangerous due to their powerful jaws and large size, it is usually advisable to treat them with drugs that are administered parenterally. However, vitamin D_3 is sufficiently effective when given orally (and since vitamin D_3 is required only one to two times weekly and in small volumes, the threat of injury is diminished!) Once the turtle is treated initially, its continued therapy can be managed via improving its diet.
iii. The aetiology of this disorder is usually a diet consisting of calcium-deficient, phosphorus-rich foodstuff, such as boneless meat and fish fillets.
iv. Change the diet to one in which calcium is readily available in the form of bone. Live fish, bone-containing flesh, etc, will furnish the necessary calcium and magnesium. Since phosphorus is present in almost everything that this species of turtle would consume, it is the one mineral that usually is not lacking in diets commonly fed to captive reptiles.

176 i. Anophthalmia.
ii. No. Eyeless or otherwise blind snakes survive well without vision; they are able to perceive prey items through chemical cues alone or, in the case of pit vipers and many boas and pythons, through the detection of warmth.
iii. Because some inbred lines of snakes appear to have a relatively high incidence of anophthalmia, this animal should not be used for breeding purposes.

177 This radiograph shows a hog-nosed snake with a distinctly and repetitively kinked vertebral spine.
i. What is your interpretation of this radiographic image?
ii. What is your tentative diagnosis of this condition?
iii. How could you confirm your diagnosis?
iv. What would be a rational treatment for this disorder?

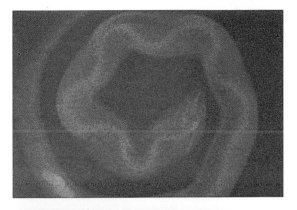

178 i. What is the shiny dark object near the midline of the plastral surface of this red-eared slider turtle?
ii. How would you treat this condition?

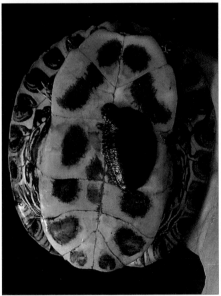

179 This ECG (lead III) is from a yellow-margined Asian box turtle that had been fed a diet of iceberg lettuce, fresh fruit, beef heart and fish fillets.
i. What is your interpretation of the ECG tracing?
ii. What is the underlying aetiology of this condition?
iii. How would you treat this condition?

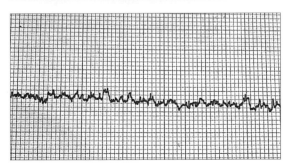

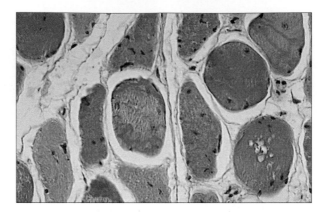

177 i. The multiple vertebral irregularities are consistent with an induced or acquired myopathy rather than a primary osseous lesion. Note that the vertebrae and ribs are smooth and free of osseous lesions; they are being pulled into angular deformation by abnormal muscular traction.
ii. Myopathy. The photomicrograph (**above**) illustrates the characteristic 'moth-eaten' appearance of some of the affected fibres from this snake's epaxial muscles.
iii. A muscle biopsy.
iv. Depending upon the type of myopathy, vitamin E (alpha- and mixed tocopherols) and selenium are worthy of a trial course of treatment.

178 i. A leech (*Placobdella* sp.).
ii. Place the turtle in a shallow container of carbonated water for a few minutes. This will cause the leech to release its hold on the turtle, and enable its easy removal.

179 i. Atrial fibrillation and first-degree heart block.
ii. Hypocalcaemia (diet together with the abnormalities revealed by the ECG).
iii. Parenteral 10% calcium gluconate or 10% calcium lactate (2.5mg/kg intracoelomically); oral administration of vitamin D_3 (1–4 iu/kg twice weekly); and a change in diet to a more calcium-rich ration containing bones, calcium carbonate, and collard, turnip or mustard greens.

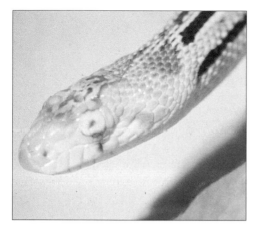

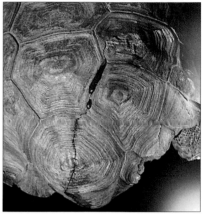

180 This adult lined-phase gopher snake has an ocular lesion. Both eyes are identically affected.
i. What is your diagnosis?
ii. What is the aetiology of this ophthalmic condition?

181 An injured desert tortoise is shown.
i. What major organs might have been injured?
ii. What are the immediate priorities?
iii. How should this be managed for the longer term?

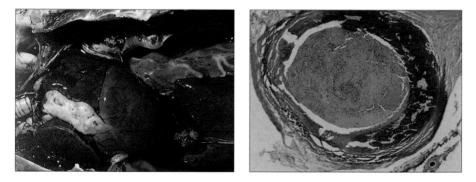

182 The cadaver of a mature common green iguana was submitted for necropsy. The diet consisted almost solely of commercial canned dog food and monkey biscuits softened with water. All of the larger arteries, trachea and pulmonary airways were found to be hard and distorted (above, left). Histopathological investigation of H&E-stained tissue sections revealed masses of red-staining material within the affected soft tissues (above, right).
i. What is your diagnosis?
ii. What was the pathogenesis of this condition?
iii. What recommendation(s) would you make to the owner of this iguana to avoid this condition with his other iguanas?

180 i. Dermatisation of the cornea and tertiary spectacle.
ii. An inheritable autosomal dominant genetic defect; therefore, affected snakes should not be used for breeding.

181 i. Lungs, kidneys, gonads and adrenal glands.
ii. Observe and treat for traumatic shock using an intravenous or intracoelomic injection of a physiological fluid, eg, Ringer's solution; if necessary, parenteral corticosteroids and a broad-spectrum antibiotic can be administered. Cleanse the wound thoroughly with 0.75% chlorhexidine solution and, after drying, stabilise the carapace with adhesive or strapping tape.
iii. Apply a supportive splint-patch constructed of one or more laminated layers of rapid-polymerising epoxy resin and steam-sterilised fibreglass cloth.

182 i. Mineralisation of soft tissues containing smooth muscle.
ii. Many, if not most, commercial dog, cat and primate foods contain high levels of vitamin D_3. Oversupplementation of reptiles with sources of vitamin D_3, together with ample calcium intake, often leads to hypervitaminosis D_3 and hypercalcaemia. The situation can be exacerbated when urinary and faecal excretion of calcium is diminished; the mineral accumulates and is often deposited in soft tissue sites, particularly those containing smooth muscle fibres. These usually involve the cardiorespiratory, alimentary and genitourinary systems, but can also include skin, skeletal muscle, and endocrine and central nervous systems.
iii. Iguanas are facultative folivores. They have evolved anatomical and physiological mechanisms for processing plant fibre by utilising hindgut fermentation. Their diets should consist of larger amounts of high-quality leafy plants and lesser amounts of fruits and animal protein. Exposing the iguana to unfiltered sunlight once or twice weekly, or furnishing the cage with an appropriate source of full-spectrum ultraviolet light will enable the iguana to synthesise its own vitamin D_3 through normal metabolic pathways.

183 This turtle is floating in a container of water with one of its sides higher than the other.
i. What is your diagnosis of the condition that is responsible for this turtle's swimming behaviour.
ii. What single diagnostic test would confirm your diagnosis?
iii. How would you treat this patient?

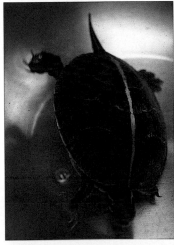

184 This radiograph is a lateral view of a rosy boa.
i. What is your tentative diagnosis?
ii. How could you confirm your diagnosis?

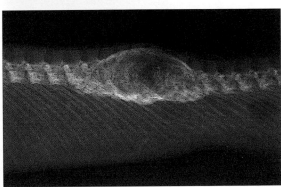

185 This Javanese file snake, or 'kurung', is a species native to an esturine habitat. Its corneas suddenly became progressively opaque within 24 hours of its being placed into an aquarium half-filled with municipal tap water.
i. What is your diagnosis?
ii. What was the aetiology of this condition?
iii. How should it be treated?
iv. What is the prognosis?

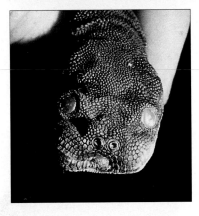

183 i. Unilateral pneumonia with loss of aeration in the left lung. The right lung is buoyant; the left lung is not. Therefore, the turtle floats with its left side submerged.
ii. Radiography will reveal the unilateral radiolucent aerated right lung field and a concomitantly radiodense left lung field.
iii. After obtaining a specimen of sputum from the pharynx, the turtle should be treated with a broad-spectrum bacteriocidal antibiotic. Keeping the turtle out of water except to drink and eat will reduce its struggling and avoid exhaustion. Often, a turtle's collapsed lung heals with scarring and does not reinflate.

184 i. Mature bone cyst and osteolysis involving the bodies and processes of 11 vertebrae.
ii. With the snake anaesthetised, perform a fine-needle aspiration of the bony mass and examine the specimen histologically. In this instance, the cystic lesion was found to be a focus of osteomyelitis that was well encapsulated by a wall composed of mature sclerotic bone.

185 i. Corneal oedema.
ii. This snake has adapted to brackish water. When placed into fresh water, the physiological 'sodium pump' failed. The corneal tissues became overhydrated and assumed a cloudy appearance.
iii. Place the snake into physiological saline solution.
iv. The tertiary spectacles and corneas soon re-establish their electrolyte balance and clear spontaneously (**below**), usually within 24 hours.

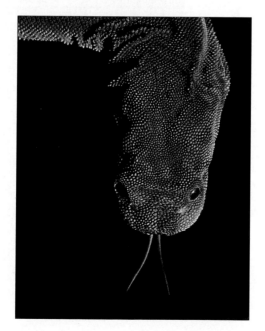

186 This necropsy specimen is of a tortoise's forelimb incised in sagittal section. The tortoise had been reluctant to walk.
i. What is your diagnosis?
ii. Had this tortoise lived, how would you have treated this condition?

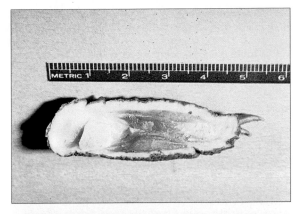

187 i. What is your diagnosis of the condition evident in this hatchling California king snake?
ii. What is the likely aetiology of this condition?
iii. How would you treat it?

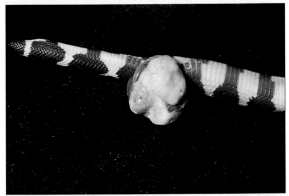

188 A map turtle during necropsy is shown.
i. What is your clinical impression of this turtle's liver?
ii. What conditions cause this kind of hepatic alteration?

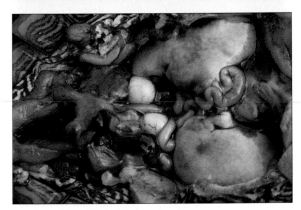

186 i. Periarticular gout.

ii. Increase the tortoise's hydration by feeding moisture-laden food – for example, soft fruit. Decrease sources of dietary animal protein. Administer allopurinol orally (10–15mg/kg daily). Allopurinol will only reduce the amount of urate salts produced by the liver; it does not diminish the urates already deposited in and around the joints and in other sites. Small (0.10–0.75mg/kg) oral doses of aspirin will provide some relief from the pain associated with gout, but may predispose the tortoise to gastrointestinal irritation and bleeding.

187 i. Prolapse of the umbilicus, yolk sac remnant and coelomic fat. Prolapse most often occurs when the fresh umbilicus adheres to a dry, unyielding surface.

ii. Shortly after hatching, the snake was placed into a cage that was lined with paper. The fresh umbilicus adhered to the paper liner and, as the hatchling tried to crawl, it partially eviscerated itself.

iii. Cleanse the prolapsed tissue; apply a ligature; excise the redundant tissue; and close the umbilical opening with two sutures.

188 i. Hydropic degeneration.

ii. Any of several metabolic disorders and chronic intoxications can induce this severe, but reversible, hepatic alteration. Hydropic degeneration commonly accompanies chronic, untreated diabetes mellitus.

189 The multiple layers of tertiary spectacle shield tissue that cover and protect the outer surface of the cornea of this snake's eye (**right**) should have been shed along with the senescent integument at each moult. These shields have been retained; this is now causing diminished visual acuity, and the retained shields can serve as a suitable habitat for parasitic mites.

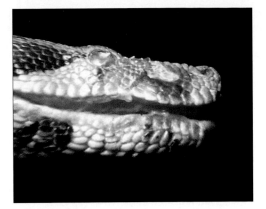

i. How would you treat this condition?

ii. What measures can you advise the owner to take to help prevent this disorder?

190 The photomicrograph (**right**) is of a merthiolate-stained wet mount made from fluid recovered from the stomach of a snake after a gastric lavage. An H&E-stained histological section of the gastric fundus from the same snake is also shown (**below, right**).

i. What is the small organism in the middle of the microscopic field in the first picture? Myriad numbers of the same organism are seen attached to the cellular borders of the gastric pits in the second picture.

ii. What is the prognosis?

iii. How would you manage this condition in a colony of snakes?

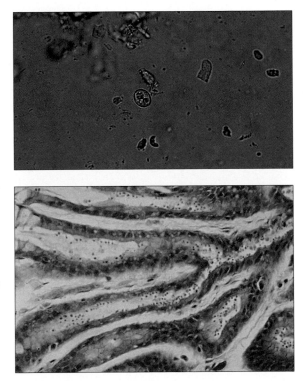

189 i. Soak the snake in mildy tepid water for at least 30 minutes. Apply one to two drops of hard contact lens wetting solution. Using a smooth-wire ear loop, gently sweep the perispectacular fornix to loosen the moisturised retained spectacles, and lift them away with a fine-pattern forceps. It is important not to apply excessive force when performing this manoeuvre.

ii. Increase the relative humidity in the snake's enclosure. Provide a suitable substrate or cage furniture upon which the snake can rub to loosen its old epidermis at the initiation of its moult. Observe the snake regularly so that remedial action can be taken before minor physical problems become serious and chronic.

190 i. *Cryptosporidium serpentis.*

ii. Very guarded to poor because, to date, there appears to be no effective treatment for this severe parasitism in reptiles; the drugs most often used to treat human cryptosporidiosis have not been effective in reptiles.

iii. (1) Identify and destroy animals which are found to be infected; (2) embargo all releases from the infected colony or collection so that potential carrier snakes do not become a threat to other collections; (3) implement strict cage decontamination and hygiene; (4) establish and adhere to a quarantine period during which adequate testing will disclose carrier snakes; and (5) test the food and water supplies for the collection to guarantee that they are free from cryptosporidial infection.

191 This organism was found in the tissues of a green sea turtle.
i. What is it?
ii. What is its major biological (and clinical) signicance?

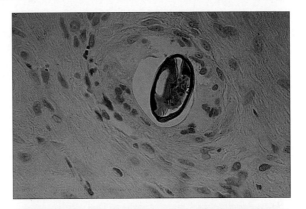

192 The plastral surface of a red-legged tortoise is shown.
i. What is the sex of this tortoise?
ii. What is the function of the plastral 'deformity' displayed by this chelonian?

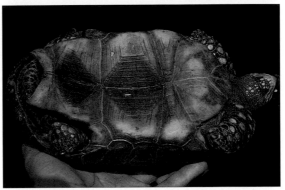

193 A Wright's-stained whole blood specimen from a wild-caught common green iguana was examined microscopically and revealed the presence of many red blood cells containing oval intraerythrocytic structures which stained pale blue.
i. What is your diagnosis?
ii. What is the significance of these intracellular objects?

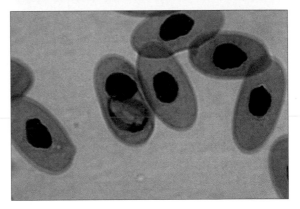

191 i. A trematode ovum.

ii. The presence of these fluke ova has been associated with fibropapillomatous tumours in marine turtles. The often exuberant neoplastic growths can create hydro-dynamic drag on these ordinarily streamlined turtles and, when present on the tur-tle's eyelids, may obscure their vision, thus making it impossible for them to find food.

192 i. Male.

ii. The deep concavity of the male tortoise's plastron matches an opposite convexity of a conspecific female tortoise's caudal carapace, thus enabling the two tortoises to copulate without the male falling to one side or another during intromission.

193 i. *Schellackia.*

ii. Although these haematoprotozoa are parasitic, they are of minimal pathogenicity unless the iguana host is immunocompromised or severely stressed. Therefore, *Schellackia* infections are not usually treated.

194 These ciliated proto-zoan microorganisms (**top, right** and **middle, right**) were found in the faeces of a Hermann's tortoise.
i. What is your diagnosis?
ii. Is the presence of these organisms significant?
iii. If so, what is the correct treatment?

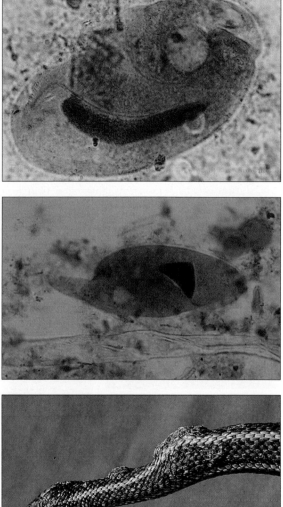

195 This Western terrestrial garter snake has multiple raised and crusted lesions on its integument. These masses have been present for almost one year.
i. What is your diagnosis?
ii. With what other kind of disorder(s) might these lesions be confused?
iii. What tests would you perform in order to narrow and then confirm the diagnosis?

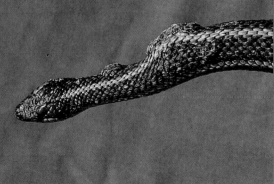

194 i. *Nyctotherus kyphoides* (**first picture**) and *Balantidium eleacus* (**second picture**).
ii. Both of these organisms are considered to be commensal microflora that are essential for the processing of cellulose into simple sugars and fatty acids.
iii. Being part of the commensal microflora, these organisms are not parasitic. Therefore, treatment is not only unnecessary, it is contraindicated.

195 i. Neoplasia.
ii. Dermatomycosis; encysted subcuticular parasites; pemphigoid dermatitis.
iii. A full-thickness skin biopsy; microbiological culture and sensitivity testing. In this case, the diagnosis was malignant chromatophoroma (mixed melanoma/erythrophoroma).

The figure **below, left** shows gross pathological specimens illustrating the diverse colouration of this tumour, ranging from orange, to red, to jet-black. The figure **below, right** is a photomicrograph of a stained section of a representative portion of this snake's chromatophoroma. Note the elongated pigment-packed tumour cells.

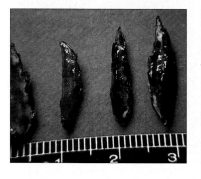 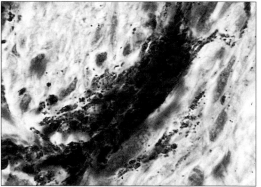

196 This stained blood film is from a rhinoceros viper.
i. What are the two cells in the centre of the image?
ii. What is the function of each type of cell?

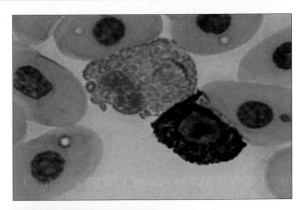

197 An iguana's mouth is shown being held open .
i. What major clinical abnormality is shown?
ii. To what organ or organs might this disorder be linked?
iii. How would you confirm your diagnosis?

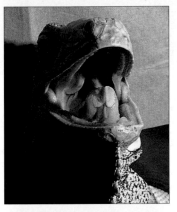

198 This whole body radiograph shows three radiopaque lesions in a desert tortoise.
i. What are these lesions?
ii. How would you treat this tortoise?

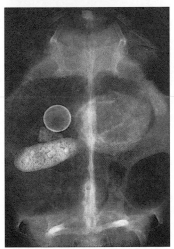

196 i. A heterophil and a basophil. Note the shapes and colours of each cell's granules.

ii. Heterophils are the reptilian counterparts of mammalian polymorphonuclear neutrophils, ie, they degranulate and release bacteriolytic enzymes. Basophils release heparin and other bioactive substances in response to complement during complement activation.

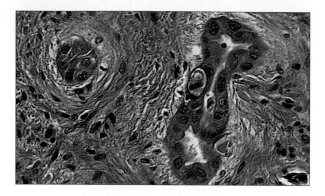

197 i. Icteric oral mucous membranes. Note: the paired white plaques are normal cartilaginous structures.

ii. Hepatic, renal, haematopoietic and reticuloendothelial systems.

iii. Biochemistry would provide evidence of hepatic and/or renal dysfunction as well as several other vital organ functions. A complete blood count would disclose the magnitude of the icterus index and erythrocytic indices, and whether erythrophagocytosis was occurring. In this case, the liver was extremely fibrotic (**above**). Only a few isolated cords of liver tissue survived compression and subsequent atrophy.

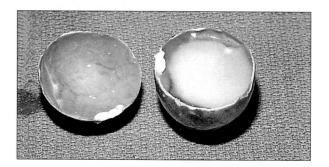

198 i. Large urolith within the urinary bladder; intraluminal spherical object with a radiopaque wall; intraluminal gravel-like foreign bodies within the intestine.

ii. Exploratory coeliotomy, urocystotomy and enterotomy to remove these radiopaque objects. During the urocystotomy a large urolith and a necrotic egg (**above**) were removed.

199 This is one of a group of juvenile red-eared slider turtles that was kept in a pet shop for several months. Suddenly, all of the turtles refused to feed. Inspection revealed that they had swollen eyes and were blowing bubbles from their mouths and external nares.
i. What is your diagnosis?
ii. What husbandry conditions are likely to have induced this disorder?
iii. How should it be treated?
iv. How can it be prevented?

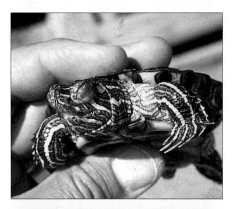

200 i. What is the cottony-white substance on this turtle's mandible and shell?
ii. How would you treat this condition?

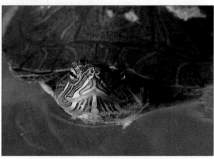

201 This necropsy specimen is of the liver removed from a long-term captive adult desert tortoise that had been fed a diet consisting of canned dog food and fresh vegetables in approximately equal parts.
i. What is your diagnosis of the condition(s) shown?
ii. What was the underlying aetiology of this disorder?
iii. How can it be prevented?

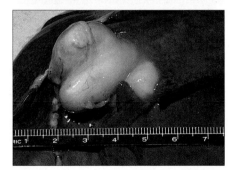

199 i. Hypovitaminosis A-induced blepharitis.
ii. A diet deficient in either beta carotene or preformed vitamin A retinol or retinyl ester, and rich in animal protein.
iii. Vitamin A or beta carotene should be administered orally. The dosage varies with the severity of the lesion, its chronicity, and whether preformed retinol (or retinyl) ester or beta carotene is used.
iv. Providing growing turtles with either a natural source of beta carotene in the form of orange, yellow and green leafy vegetables, or living algae, or supplementing their diet with an oral source of preformed vitamin A in the form of a commercial product specifically formulated for semi-aquatic turtles.

200 i. Saprolegniasis.
ii. Soak affected turtles in 1.0% chlorhexidine solution or malachite green/dilute formalin solution for 30 minutes daily for five to seven consecutive days. Keep the turtles dry except when they are being fed and watered, or being treated with the protocol recommended. When the turtles are being kept dry, their integument should be painted or sprayed with full-strength povidone iodine solution which is permitted to dry on the epidermal surfaces.

201 i. Cholecystolithiasis (**below, left**) and cholecytitis (**below, right**).
ii. Desert tortoises are largely facultative herbivores; in their natural habitat, their diet consists mostly of vegetable matter. Regularly feeding herbivorous reptiles a fat-laden item, such as canned dog food, will yield an unnatural diet that is composed of too much animal protein and lipid, promoting inflammation of the gall bladder and the formation of gallstones. In addition, many commercial dog, cat and primate diets contain high levels of vitamins A and D_3. Therefore, it is common to find lesions of smooth muscle mineralisation in herbivorous reptiles fed these inappropriate dietary items.

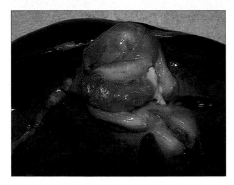
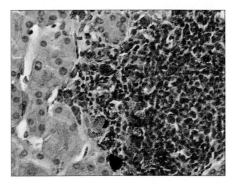

202 i. What is the condition illustrated in the oral cavities of these two boa constrictors (**top, right** and **middle, right**)?
ii. What is the aetiology?
iii. How should it be treated?

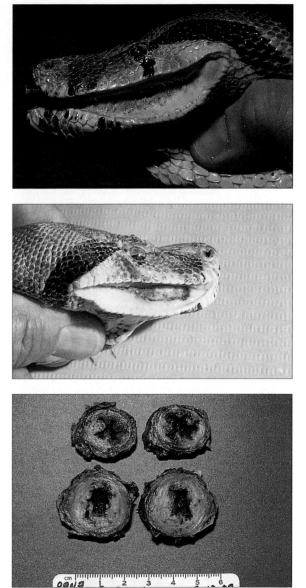

203 Four sections of the large intestine from a mature boa constrictor at necropsy are shown.
i. From the gross alterations exhibited in these specimens, what is your diagnosis?
ii. Which common protozoan parasite is most likely to have caused this lesion?
iii. When diagnosed sufficiently early, which chemotherapeutic agents are effective in treating this?

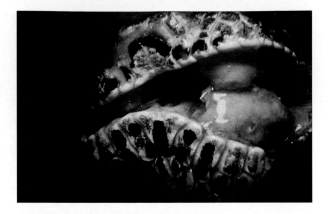

202 i. Ulcerative stomatitis ('mouth rot').
ii. A wide variety of Gram-negative and Gram-positive microorganisms can cause this type of lesion, although Gram-negative pathogens are most often isolated. The snake shown in the first picture yielded *Aeromonas hydrophila*; the snake shown in the second yielded *Klebsiella* sp. A more advanced case of ulcerative (and pyogranulomatous) stomatitis from which *Morganella morgani* and *Proteus vulgaris* were cultured in large numbers is illustrated (**above**).
iii. The oral tissues should be cleansed gently with dilute hydrogen peroxide, chlorhexidine, or povidone iodine solution. Once the mucosae are free of exudate, the affected tissues should be covered with an appropriate antibiotic ointment or cream. Parenteral antibiotics should also be administered. Physiological fluids should be administered daily (20–25ml/kg) in order to maintain fluid balance and renal perfusion, and to prevent accumulation of potentially toxic antibiotic(s).

203 i. Intestinal entamoebiasis.
ii. *Entamoeba invadens.*
iii. Colubrid snakes should be treated with metronidazole (40mg/kg, repeated after two weeks); Boidae, Viperidae and Elapidae require 125–250mg/kg. Antibiotic therapy, fluid replacement, and compassionate supportive nursing care are necessary treatments for this serious protozoan infection, because snakes (and other reptiles) infected with *E. invadens* are often extremely ill and labile.

204 i. Identify the ophthalmic condition evident in this immature musk turtle's eye.
ii. What would your treatment be for this condition?
iii. How does the treatment differ from the treatment of the identical disorder in a dog or cat?

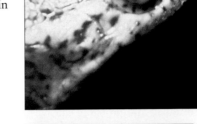

205 The gross *post-mortem* appearance of a female emydid turtle is shown.
i. What is your diagnosis?
ii. What is the likely aetiology for this condition?

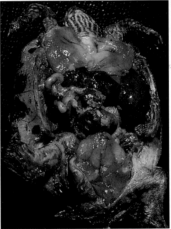

206 This female western toad sustained a crushing injury to its left hindlimb that resulted in an open, comminuted femoral fracture and considerable soft tissue trauma and maceration.
i. How would you manage this case?
ii. Would it be humane to release this toad after treatment?

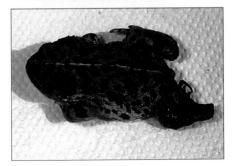

204 i. Anterior uveitis.
ii. Topical instillation of a mydriatic, a broad-spectrum bacteriocidal antibiotic, and corticosteroids; if necessary, parenteral antibiotics also can be administered.
iii. Because of the presence of striated muscle fibres in reptilian and amphibian irides, d-tubocurarine is instilled into the eye to dilate the pupil rather than homatropine.

205 i. Severe chronic yolk-induced serocoelomitis.
ii. Exposure of the coelom to free egg yolk resulting from laceration or rupture of the oviduct and spillage of lipid-rich yolk into the cavity.

206 i. The left hindlimb is irreparably damaged and should be amputated. The devitalised and grossly contaminated tissue may cause further harm to normal tissues and structures, particularly intracoelomic organs which lie immediately beneath and adjacent to the crushed limb. Rather than leave a truncated stump that would only become abraded and probably chronically infected, the femur should be disarticulated and the surgical incision closed with synthetic absorbable sutures. A light covering of an antiseptic liquid plastic bandage helps keep the incision dry and clean, thus permitting rapid and complete healing to take place (**below**).

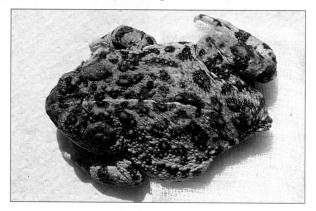

ii. It would be entirely humane to release this toad after the incision had healed because toads ambulate by crawling rather than by jumping; they learn quickly to crawl quite well on their three remaining limbs. Also, since toads' skin secretes toxic substances, these animals have relatively few predators.

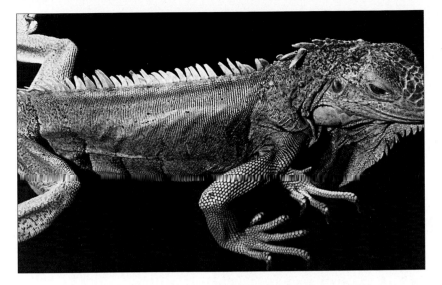

207 A mature male common iguana was presented with a history of severe and chronic weight loss and muscle atrophy. It still had an appetite, and had been fed high-calcium, low-phosphorus green leafy vegetables and fresh ripe fruits. The faeces had been soft, but mostly formed, and a faecal examination was negative for parasites and ova. The haemogram and physiologic chemistries (except for plasma protein) were within the normal range published for this species. Specifically, the blood glucose was 122mg/dl; glucose was not detected in the urine. Plasma protein was 2.3mg/dl with a globulin fraction of 1.8mg/dl and an albumin of 0.5mg/dl. The liver-specific enzyme profile was normal. Oral mucous membranes were pink. Except for a mildly osteopenic radiographic appearance to its skeleton, there were no radiographic abnormalities. Doppler ultrasonic blood-flow investigation revealed grade IV/VI atrioventricular and aortic murmurs radiating bilaterally outward to the brachiocephalic, carotid, and subclavian arteries. Because the iguana was so profoundly thin and cachectic, euthanasia was carried out and a necropsy performed. The only gross pathologic abnormalities noted were a total lack of body fat, diffusely atrophic skeletal muscles, accentuated small and large intestinal mucosal pattern, a very small liver, small and soft testes, and mildly soft cranial bones which incised with minimal resistance. What are some alternative diagnoses?

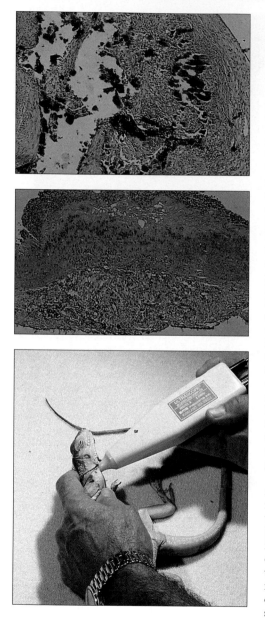

207 The correct diagnosis was protein-wasting enteropathy. Histopathology revealed non-suppurative enteritis, valvular endocardiosis, and polyarterial medial mineralisation. Alternative *ante-mortem* diagnoses could be: chronic pancreatic and/or hepatic insufficiency, intracoelomic neoplasia, muscular dystrophy, nephrosis, intoxication, intussusception, parasitic cyst(s), severe gastrointestinal parasitism, and pyogranulomatosis. Several potential diagnoses can be discarded because analyses for enteric (intraluminal) parasitism, hypo- and hyperglycaemia, and hepatic dysfunction do not support these diagnoses. Icterus was not evident clinically since the iguana's plasma was clear and not yellow. The loud valvular murmurs were probably caused by both the widespread endocardiosis and the relatively low-viscosity blood due to hypoproteinaemia. The iguana's liver was able to synthesize protein, but the diffuse inflammatory bowel disease was permitting substantial amounts of protein (and other nutrients) to be lost in the stools. Note that the plasma protein was very depressed, and that the little protein that was produced was mostly attributable to the globulin fraction.

Note the extreme thinness and muscle atrophy of this iguana. The necropsy examination revealed a variably thick-walled, inflamed large bowel filled with liquid faeces. The figure **top, left** is a photomicrograph of the massively mineralised aorta of this lizard (H & E, x27 original magnification). The **middle** figure shows one of the heart valves illustrating the severe inflammation that was found in this iguana. The **lower** figure illustrates the use of a Doppler ultrasonic blood-flow detector in a young iguana.

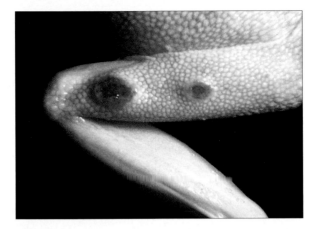

208 This amelanistic tree frog exhibits two integumentary lesions on the inner surface of its right hindleg.
i. What is your diagnosis?
ii. What organisms are likely to be associated with such a lesion?

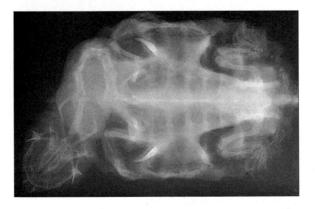

209 What are the bilateral, sharply pointed and angulated osseous structures found in the anterior cervical region of the radiograph of this mature female mata mata turtle?

208 i. Ulcerative dermatitis, a subacute form of 'red-leg.'
ii. *Aeromonas hydrophila, A. aerogenes, A. aerophila, A. salmonicida, Pseudomonas* spp., *Klebsiella* spp., *Morganella* spp., *Proteus* spp., etc.

209 The sharply angled bones are part of the hyoid apparatus which supports the lingual musculature and enables this aquatic side-necked turtle to literally 'vacuum' the fish upon which it subsists into its very large mouth.

The figure **below** is of a living mata mata turtle. Note the snorkel-like proboscis, broad mouth, and bright pink chin skin that characterise this largely aquatic and highly-prized chelonian.

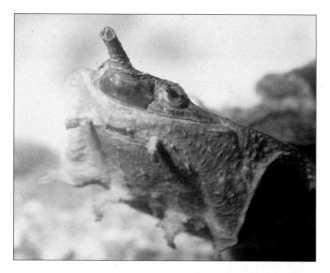

210 This arthropod was found on a corn snake housed in a cage furnished with aspen wood 'wool'.
i. What is this creature?
ii. Is it parasitic?
iii. What is its significance?

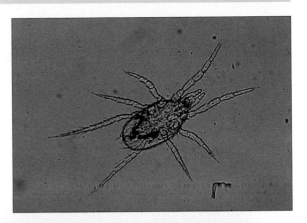

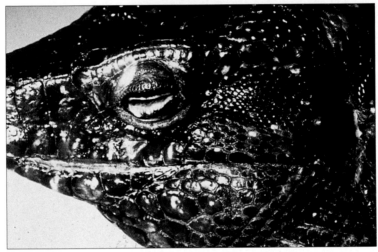

211 This mature red tegu lizard (**above**) had been fed a diet of killed, frozen, then thawed mice and small rats. It presented with a chronic skin condition characterised by the retention of skin that should have been sloughed. The result of this failure to moult its skin was a greatly thickened and hyperkeratotic integument that could not be peeled even after prolonged soaking in warm water and repeated application of keratolytic agents.
i. What factors contributed to this condition?
ii. How is this condition best treated?

210 i. An adult trombiculid grain mite.

ii. The adult stage of this mite is not parasitic; only the nymphal stage, which can be readily identified because it has only three pairs of legs, is parasitic. The adults are free living and feed upon organic dust particles.

iii. The immature stages will parasitise vertebrates in their environment, and the cage litter used in the corn snake's cage was infested before it was placed into the cage.

211 i. This case of hypovitaminosis A was induced by the high-protein diet that was fed to this usually omnivorus species of lizard. In their native habitat, tegu lizards eat small mammals, birds, other lizards, eggs, carrion and ripe fruit that they scavenge on the ground. Vitamin A is required in order to metabolise protein and maintain epithelial surfaces.

ii. Oral administration of vitamin A injected into the tegu's dead mice or rat prey (1,000IU/carcase). The tegu was fed four to six mice or two medium-sized rats weekly and, in addition, it was fed cooked, mashed yellow and orange squash, pumpkin and sweet potatoes, plus fresh kiwi fruit and berries. Providing these large lizards with a water container deep enough to bathe in helps soften the skin sufficiently to permit them to moult without retaining skin 'tags' which often accumulate on the digits and tail.

212 i. What is your diagnosis of the condition afflicting this adult male red-legged tortoise?
ii. How would you treat this condition?

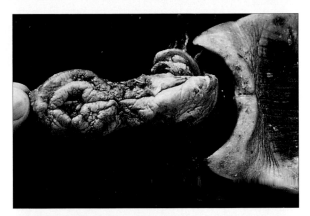

213 This 26-year-old South American boa constrictor has been on display in a professional collection all her life and is eating well and acting normally.
i. What ophthalmic conditions are evident?
ii. How would you manage this case?

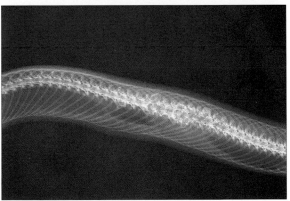

214 A copperhead snake is presented for examination because it is not crawling normally. There is no history of trauma. What does the radiograph reveal?

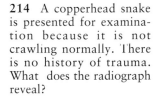

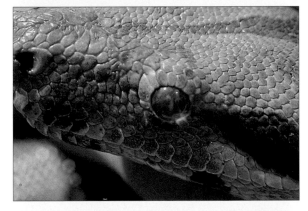

212 i. Chronic prolapse and maceration of the penis.
ii. The tissue is obviously devitalised and the penis is paralysed. Therefore, anaesthetise the tortoise, retract the penis, place through-and-through transfixing ligatures, amputate the penis distal to the ligatures, and permit the stump to retract into the cloaca.

213 i. Lenticular cataracts and glaucoma. Both lenses exhibited opacification. Slit-lamp ophthalmoscopy revealed glaucoma in one eye.
ii. This snake was not treated for either of these ophthalmic disorders because there was no evidence of discomfort and the cataracts were not causing the snake any problems. Also, the impermeable tertiary spectacles made it virtually impossible for ophthalmic drops or ointments to be used topically. In consultation with the snake's owner, the boa will be permitted to live out her life until she shows signs of pain or disability.

214 Multifocal osteolytic and osteoproductive lesions affecting the vertebral bodies and spinous processes and, to a lesser extent, the ribs. These characteristics are more consistent with osteomyelitis and pyogranulomatous osteitis, rather than with osteitis deformans (Paget's disease of bone) which is usually marked by a more exuberant osteoproliferative reaction. In this instance, the histopathologically-confirmed diagnosis was pyogranulomatous (largely histiocytic) bacterial osteitis and osteomyelitis.

215 This adult Solomon Island prehensile-tail skink has a slowly growing proliferative mass arising from its mandible that has been present for three months.
i. What are your differential diagnoses?
ii. How would you confirm the diagnosis?
iii. What is your treatment?

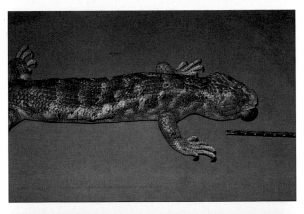

216 The intermandibular (gular) region of a Burmese python is shown.
i. What is your diagnosis?
ii. What is the significance of this condition?

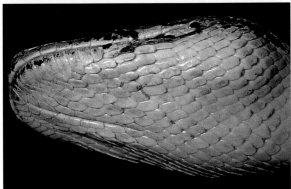

217 What does the lateral projection radiograph of the spinal column of this mature iguana reveal?

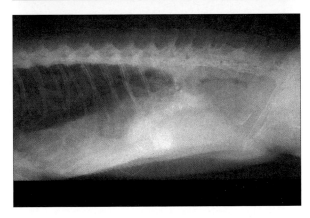

215 i. Neoplasia and chronic inflammation.
ii. Fine-needle or wedge biopsy with microbiological culture, stained cytology and histopathological examination of stained microsections.
iii. Biopsy revealed a multilocular granuloma from which *Seratia marcescens* was cultured. The highly vascular mass was excised, and the exposed bed treated with three freeze-thaw cycles of cryosurgery using liquid nitrogen. Intramuscular enrofloxacin (7.5mg/kg daily) was given.

216 i. Multiple subepidermal haemorrhages.
ii. Septicaemia. This python had a severe disseminated *Klebsiella* infection with multi-organ involvement. It was treated aggressively with a bacteriocidal antibiotic, and given fluid therapy and supportive nursing.

217 Ossifying spondylosis of the thoracolumbar vertebra. This is a relatively common inflammatory lesion found in captive green iguanas. If the lesions are solitary and if pathological fractures do not develop, they are of minimal clinical significance and appear to be part of the ageing process in these long-lived lizards.

218 The integument of this collared lizard has a red-orange mass on its surface.
i. What is your diagnosis?
ii. What is its significance?
iii. How would you treat this condition?

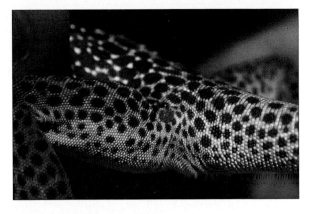

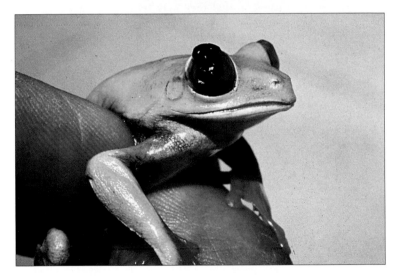

219 This is one of several red-eyed frogs that presented with eye trauma with deep multifocal laceration to their corneas which, in some instances, could lead to iris prolapse. The frogs were kept in a terrarium furnished with living tropical plants, and they were fed live domestic crickets *ad libidum* (the crickets had foraged upon whatever organic matter was available in the terrarium).
i. What is your diagnosis?
ii. What advice would you give to the owner in order to avoid this condition?

218 i. Infestation with the trombiculid lizard mite, *Herstiella trombidiiformis*. Note the pointed protruberance at the caudal end of the mite's abdomen; the presence of this structure helps differentiate this mite from *Ophionyssus natricis*.

ii. These ectoparasites cause local irritation induced by their bites and, therefore, provide an entry for pathogens into the irritated and inflamed integument. If large numbers of these mites are present, they can induce severe blood-loss anaemia.

iii. Masses of these mites can be removed with a cotton-tipped applicator that has been moistened in an insecticide formulated to be safe for young puppies and kittens. After the masses of mites have been removed, the infested lizard should be wiped down with a cotton sponge barely moistened with the same insecticide. Lastly, the cage and all of its 'furniture' must be either discarded or thoroughly cleansed to eradicate any residual mites or their ova.

219 i. Cricket-induced trauma to the corneas resulting in an iris prolapse (**below**).

ii. Limit the number of crickets that are offered as prey, or provide food for any crickets that escape being eaten so that they may feed upon something other than their erstwhile predators. Also, it is wise to inspect the inhabitants of any terrarium frequently so that if problems arise, they can be resolved quickly.

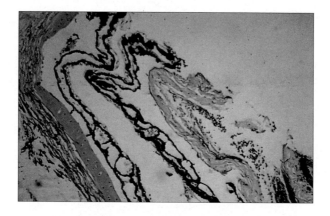

220 These flagellated organisms were recovered from a mosquito that had fed upon an infected fence lizard. What are they?

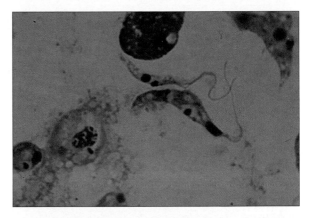

221 This juvenile green iguana has a massively swollen left hindlimb. It had sustained a severe bite from a larger male iguana two months prior to being presented for examination.
i. What is your diagnosis?
ii. How would you treat this iguana?

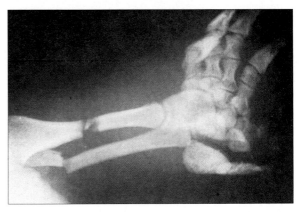

222 How would you manage the tibial and fibular fractures of the tortoise's limb illustrated in this radiograph?

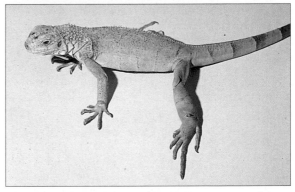

220 Trypanosomes. These haemoprotozoa are pathogenic in their reptilian hosts.

221 i. Chronic abscessation and myositis.
ii. Anaesthetise the iguana and perform a coxofemoral amputation of the entire affected limb. In this instance, the limb infection was treated aggressively because of the chronicity and because the limb was swollen so firmly. The surgical specimen depicted (below) shows the abundant dense fibrocollagenous connective tissue which surrounds the focus of infection. This dense tissue greatly impedes the distribution of an effective minimum inhibitory concentration (MIC) of antibiotic to the areas of infection. A high amputation was elected so that no stump would remain to be traumatised by the iguana treading upon it. The iguana made a rapid and complete recovery and was not particularly handicapped by the loss of its hindlimb.

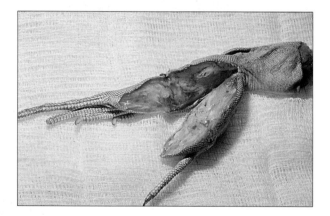

222 Because of the very limited access to the limb for the placement of intramedullary pins and the inadvisability of placing intramedullary pins in a retrograde direction from a plantar approach, this case could best be managed by using a Kirchner-Ehmer apparatus with cold-setting acrylic covering the pins and connecting rods. The limb was held in extension by placing a bulky cotton pad into the 'pocket' from which the limb exited from beneath the overhanging carapacial shell. If the tortoise had been larger, human paediatric finger plates and bone screws could have been employed in this repair. External coaptation splintage could possibly have been used, but that method was deemed inferior to this more positive approach.

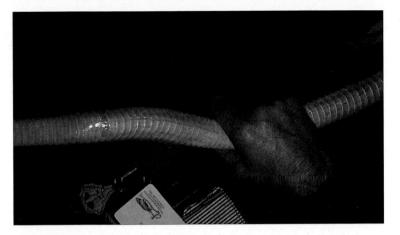

223 An Australian taipan, one of the world's most deadly venomous snakes, has a swelling in the region of its heart that is progressively growing so large that swallowing is becoming difficult. Doppler ultrasonic blood-flow detection does not reveal abnormal valvular or vascular sounds.
i. What is your tentative diagnosis?
ii. What tests or other procedures would you perform to confirm your diagnosis?

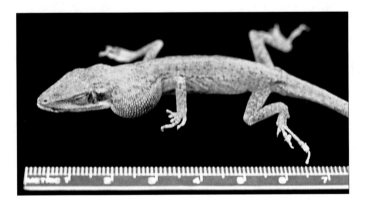

224 This adult male Carolina anole lizard has a pronounced swelling involving the left cervical region.
i. What are your tentative diagnoses?
ii. What tests or procedures would you perform to confirm your diagnosis?
iii. How would you treat this case?

223 i. Cardiomyopathy.

ii. An ECG would help differentiate electrical conduction disturbances; a radiograph would reveal the overall size and shape of the heart and disclose the presence of mineralised foci; ultrasonography would demonstrate the size, shape and function of the two atria and single ventricle in real time. In this instance, the diagnosis was cardiomyopathy arising from multiple foci of infection from which *Pseudomonas aeruginosa* was cultured. It is interesting that in this case the heart sounds arising from blood flow through the heart and over the heart valves were normal; thus, it can be inferred that vegetative endocarditis was not present.

224 i. Ascessation, pyogranulomatosis, mycetoma, neoplasia, parasitic cyst, parotid adenitis, haematoma, etc.

ii. Fine-needle aspiration biopsy, followed by cytology, histopathology, and microbiological culture and sensitivity testing. In this case, the mass was a mycetoma.

iii. Under general anaesthesia the mass should be incised and the contents removed. The cavity resulting from this excision is reduced by excising any redundant skin. The incision is not sutured, but the wound should be flushed twice daily with dilute (0.75%) chlorhexidine solution until it heals. A specific antifungal agent can also be instilled.

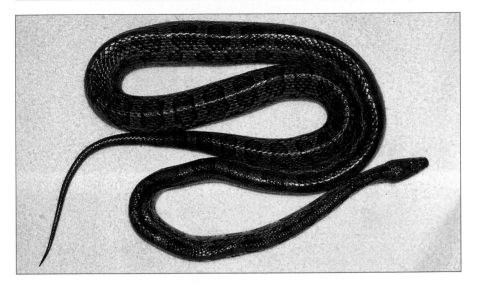

225 This 10-year-old female corn snake had been healthy and feeding on laboratory mice until three weeks prior to being presented with sudden weight loss, anorexia, cachexia and diffuse swellings.
i. What are your tentative diagnoses?
ii. What tests or procedures would you perform to confirm your diagnosis?

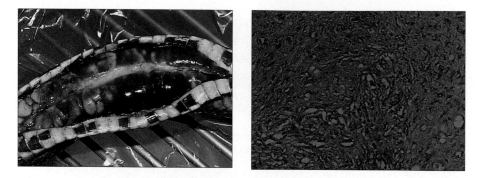

225 i. Tentative *ante-mortem* diagnoses include: chronic enteritis, yolk serocoelomitis, salpingitis, gastric cryptosporidiosis, intussusception, pyogranulomatosis, and intracoelomic neoplasia.

ii. Obtain a specimen of blood for haematology and chemistry investigation; radiograph the snake, looking for radiologically apparent abnormalities; use ultrasonography to investigate the diffuse swellings; and obtain a fine-needle biopsy of any masses. This snake died. At necropsy many viscera were found to be covered by a variably thick layer of tissue which penetrated into the affected viscera. A portion of the coelomic contents is shown (**above, left**). Histopathology revealed the abnormal tissue comprised markedly pleomorphic, multipolar, or occasionally spindyloid, cells which formed into eddy-like swirls and whorls that infiltrated, compressed and distorted normal structures (**above, right**). Other areas contained more regularly arranged sheets of cells with hyperchromatic nuclei. Binucleate and multipolar cells were occasionally observed. The edges of some areas of the mass possessed a papillary appearance. One feature consistently observed in each section of the mass was the large number of variable-sized clear clefts and round spaces lined by thin, dark-staining cells. In other portions of the mass, 'signet-ring'-shaped round spaces predominated. Because of their often poorly differentiated nature, some mesotheliomata can be particularly difficult to diagnose with absolute certainty. When examined only as H&E-stained sections, they may resemble adenocarcinomata. However, when a specific antibody linked to immunoperoxidase reagent is incubated with suspected mesotheliomatous tumour tissue sections, the specific antibody binds to its complementary antigen present in the tumour tissue. The peroxidase catalyses peroxide in the incubation medium and yields a strong cell antigen-specific reaction whose product is enhanced with chromagen reagent. The following tests and reactions are characteristic of these kinds of neoplasm, and the results of tissue sections from this tumour.

	Mesothelioma	Adenocarcinoma	Snake tumour
Alcian blue	+	–	+
Colloidal iron	+	–	+
Keratin	+	–	+
Carcinoembryonic antigen	–	+	–

Thus, as in malignant mesothelioma in 'higher' animals, the neoplasm in this snake was strongly positive for keratin, colloidal iron, and Alcian blue-staining mucopolysaccharide (probably hyaluronic acid), which is characteristic of mesothelioma; it was negative for carcinoembryonic antigen (CEA).

226 i. What does the dorsoventral radiograph of this chuckwalla lizard reveal?
ii. How would you treat this lizard?

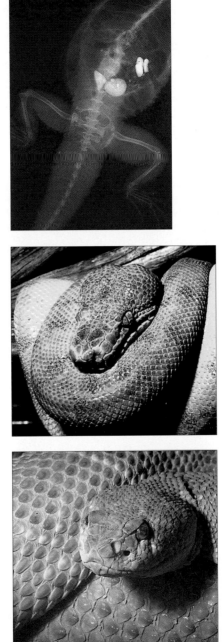

227 Some pythons and boas, and all pit vipers, possess either labial or facial pit organs. Examples are shown here (**right** and **below**). What is the function of these structures?

226 i. A markedly swollen thigh, osteolysis involving the right ilium and ischium, and multiple radiopaque foreign objects in the alimentary tract. The soft-tissue swelling and osteolysis are consistent with a diagnosis of abscessation, myositis, and osteomyelitis. The gastrointestinal foreign bodies are more radiodense than is typical of gastroliths or enteroliths and, therefore, are interpreted as being ingested stones. Although these objects are seen immediately when viewing the radiograph, they are incidental to the much more significant inflammatory bone and skeletal muscle lesions.

ii. The severe osteomyelitis, myositis, and abscessation must be treated aggressively by incision, debridement and currettage, and broad-spectrum bacteriocidal antibiotic therapy accompanied by supportive nursing care.

227 Labial and facial pits are sensitive to infrared (thermal) radiation. These special sense organs help those snakes which have them to find their warm-blooded prey and, to a lesser extent, become aware of potential warm-blooded predators. The neural signals from these structures are processed in the brain's optic centres in a fashion similar to how visual signals are processed from the eyes.

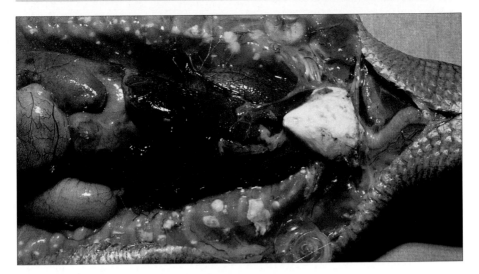

228 A juvenile Solomon Island prehensile-tailed skink dies suddenly without displaying signs of illness. During necropsy examination of the carcase, white deposits are found within the pericardial sac and beneath the serosal surfaces of the thoracic portion of the coelomic cavity.
i. What is your diagnosis?
ii. To what metabolic process(es) are these lesions related?

229 In this gecko's eye the iris has multiple pupillary apertures. This type of pupil imparts particularly acute vision in subdued illumination and, thus, is especially valuable to a lizard that hunts its prey at night. Why is the topical application of atropine sulphate or homatropine ineffective in inducing mydriasis when performing an ophthalmoscopic examination upon a reptile's eye?

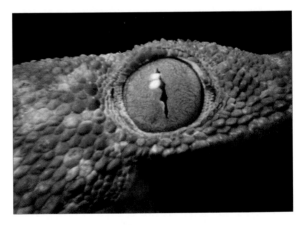

228 i. Visceral gout.

ii. Hyperuricaemia due to overwhelming the renal threshold for uric acid clearance can be induced by dehydration, a diet too high in animal protein sources, nephrosis and nephritis, and renal damage induced by nephrotoxic drugs.

229 Reptiles, like birds, have skeletal (striated) muscle tissues in their iris. This renders parasympatholytics, such as atropine or tropicamide, or sympathomimetics like phenylephrine, ineffective in producing mydriasis. Intracameral D-tubocurarine has been suggested to give local neuromuscular blockade with attendant mydriasis. Topical vecuronium is also effective, but is inappropriate in snakes and Tokay geckos where drug penetration does not occur across the spectacle.

230 What is the condition affecting the erythrocytes from a rattlesnake (**above, right**) and a Reeve's turtle (**middle, right**)?

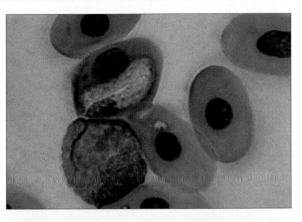

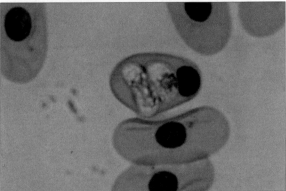

231 The owner of an Asian red-tailed rat snake is concerned because his snake's eyes have suddenly assumed a bluish, milky hue. Otherwise, the snake appears to be healthy.
i. What is your diagnosis?
ii. What is the significance of this condition?

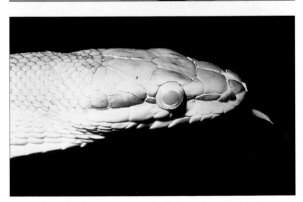

230 Haemogregarine infection. Generally, these intraerythrocytic parasites are not particularly pathogenic and, thus, their presence is not a cause for concern.

231 i. This snake is about to moult its epidermis.
ii. It is an entirely normal condition seen just prior to a skin moult.
The figure **below** illustrates the freshly moulted epidermis of a snake. As the time approaches for ecdysis to occur, a water-soluble oily substance is secreted which facilitates loosening of the old epidermis from the surface of the new integument. Once the old epidermis is detached from around the rostrum and lips, the snake crawls out of its old 'skin' and, as it does so, the outer layer is cast off and turned inside-out.

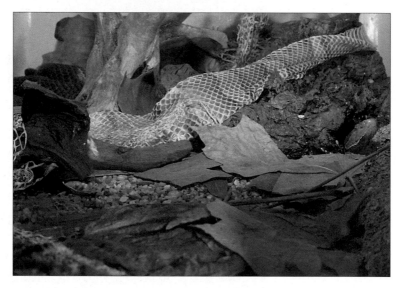

232 The dorsoventral radiograph (**above, right**) is of a half-grown Western painted turtle. The craniocaudal radiograph of the same turtle is also shown (**middle, right**).
i. What is your diagnosis?
ii. How would you treat the turtle for this condition?
iii. What is the prognosis?

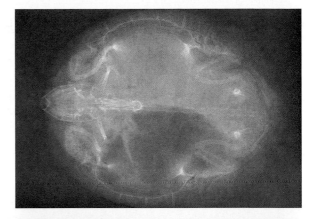

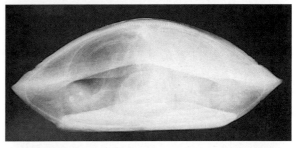

233 This semi-aquatic freshwater turtle exhibits an abnormality involving its plastron.
i. What is this abnormality?
ii. What might have caused this condition?

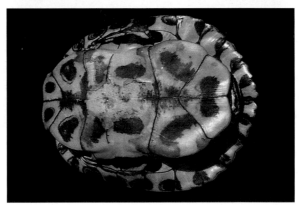

171

232 i. Unilateral and complete collapse of the left lung.

ii. Broad-spectrum bacteriocidal antibiotic therapy and supportive nursing care are required. The turtle should either be kept dry, except when being fed or permitted to drink, or it must be provided with a place onto which it can 'haul-out' of the water to rest.

iii. Unfavourable. Although the infection that caused the complete consolidation of the left lung may be brought under control, it is doubtful whether the affected lung will ever reinflate. Also, severely pneumonic lungs often heal by 'walling off' infection. This is manifested as abscesses and pyogranulomata which constitute foci for future infection to become re-established.

233 i. Subepidermal haemorrhages.

ii. Trauma, coagulopathy or infection. In this instance, the multifocal red lesions are ecchymotic haemorrhages; the turtle was thrombocytopaenic.

234 Portions of the backs of two sibling juvenile amelanistic corn snakes (whose parents were related) are shown. Both snakes appeared normal until they were six months old; then they simultaneously exhibited an identical 'lumpy bumpy' appearance.
i. What is your diagnosis?
ii. What is the underlying aetiology?

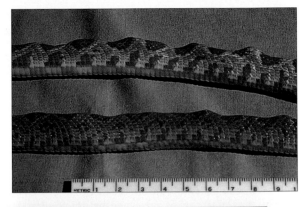

235 What is the sex of this emydid turtle?

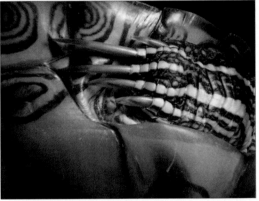

236 This radiograph shows the dorsal thoracic portion of the coelomic cavity of a young adult iguana.
i. What is your diagnosis?
ii. What is the likely cause of this lesion?
iii. What is the treatment for this condition?
iv. How can this disorder be prevented?

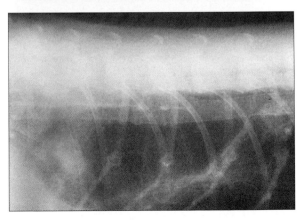

234 i. Osseous dysplasia.
ii. The disorder appears to have been due to an inherited genetic defect.

235 Male. Note the elongated claws which are a secondary sexual characteristic of male emydid turtles.

236 i. Mineralisation of the aorta and intrapulmonary airways.
ii. Iatrogenic hypercalcaemia secondary to hypervitaminosis D_3.
iii. Hypercalcaemia can be treated effectively by administering calcitonin (1.5iu/kg s/c daily) and intracoelomic Ringer's saline (15ml/kg daily). Treatment continues until the plasma calcium returns to normal (approximately 12mg/dl). The source of vitamin D_3 should be removed from the diet.
iv. This condition can be prevented by not feeding commercial dog, cat or primate food to folivorous lizards. The correct diet should include items which naturally furnish adequate calcium and other nutrients so that supplementation with vitamin-mineral products is not necessary.

237 Note the red lesion on this tree frog's rostrum, and its extreme depression. The photograph was taken just before the frog died.
i. What is your diagnosis?
ii. How do you explain the integumentary lesion and the depression?

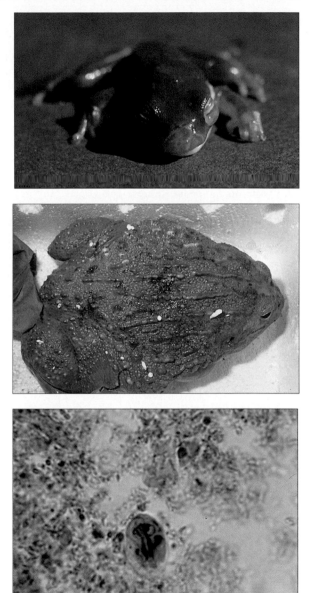

238 This African bullfrog has sustained several deep lacerations and abrasions on its dorsum and head. How would you treat this frog?

239 This photomicrograph is of a trichrome-stained organism found in the faeces of an iguana.
i. What is your diagnosis?
ii. Is this organism pathogenic?
iii. If pathogenic, how would you treat this organism?
iv. What advice would you give the owner?

237 i. Ulcerative dermatitis; subacute 'red-leg.' (Even though the major lesion is on this frog's rostrum [nose], the vernacular term 'red-leg' is used by many hobbyists to describe this septicemic disease in amphibians.)
ii. Ulcerative dermatitis in amphibians is usually caused by any of several Gram-negative bacterial pathogens, especially *Aeromonas* spp. These microorganisms are often characterised by their potent endotoxins. These infections tend to become widely disseminated and septicaemic, often affecting many vital organs simultaneously. Affected amphibians become profoundly ill and may display signs of toxic shock immediately before they die.

238 Flush the open lacerations and abrasions thoroughly with 0.75% chlorhexidine solution before applying two or more applications of a liquid plastic wound bandage, eg, Opsite, to the denuded area. This is generally preferable to suturing lacerations like these in amphibians, and it is not necessary to anaesthetise the amphibian. As the tissue heals, the plastic bandage is displaced and loosened, and eventually falls away leaving a healing scar beneath.

239 i. *Giardia lamblia*. Note the twin eye-like anterior nuclei that characterise this organism.
ii. Yes, particularly in stressed, immunocompromised patients, or in patients with other serious medical conditions.
iii. Treatment consists of metronidazole (125–250mg/kg orally every 48–72 hours for one to two weeks).
iv. Because *Giardia* can infect humans, great care must be taken to avoid faecal contamination of foodstuffs, food-preparation areas and utensils, and/or domestic water supplies.

240 This red-eared slider turtle appears to have a misshapen head.
i. What is your diagnosis?
ii. How would you treat this condition?

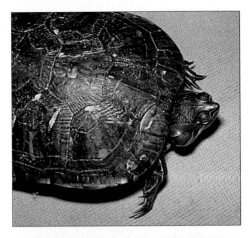

241 A Chilean tortoise is shown during a routine necropsy examination.
i. What gross alterations are displayed?
ii. Could other tortoises living within the same environment from which this tortoise came be jeopardised?

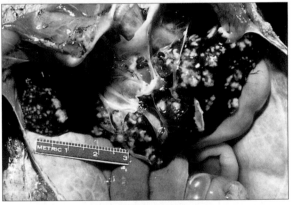
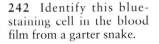

242 Identify this blue-staining cell in the blood film from a garter snake.

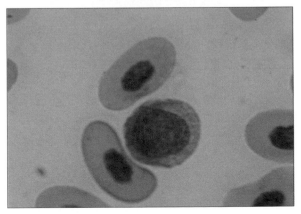

240 i. An abscess or pyogranuloma in the right parotid area.
ii. Generally, an anaesthetic is unnecessary because the treatment does not inflict severe pain. Cleanse the integument covering the mass with surgical antiseptic soap; incise over the greater curvature of the abscess down to the level of the necrotic cellular debris filling the expanded cavity, and remove the contents completely; flush the cavity with dilute chlorhexidine or dilute povidone iodine solution. Repeat twice daily until healed. Parenteral bacteriocidal antibiotics may be used as well, depending on the seriousness of the condition.

241 i. Multifocal hepatic abscessation/pyogranulomatosis.
ii. Yes. *Mycobacterium ulcerans* was isolated in pure culture from these lesions.

242 Lymphocyte.

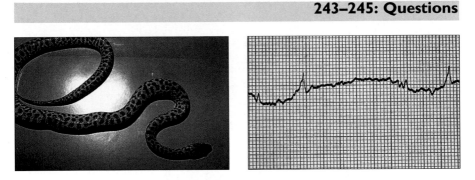

243 A Children's python (**above, left**) was presented for examination so that a progressive swelling in the region of its heart could be evaluated. A portion of the ECG from this snake is reproduced (**above, right**).
i. What are your differential diagnoses?
ii. How do you interpret the ECG?

244 These four parasites were found in the lung of a captive reticulated python.
i. What are they?
ii. What is an effective treatment for this condition?

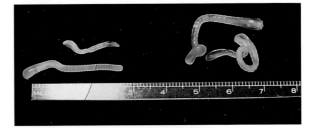

245 i. What does the dorsoventral whole-body radiograph of this Texas tortoise reveal?
ii. How would you treat this tortoise?
iii. What is a likely cause for this disorder?

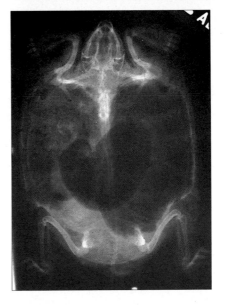

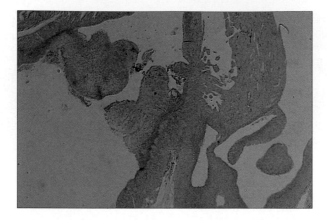

243 i. (1) Cardiomyopathy; (2) an abscess or large pyogranuloma; (3) a neoplasm; or (4) a parasitic cyst etc.
ii. The ECG exhibits first degree heart block and atrial fibrillation. The python was euthanised. The necropsy and histopathological examinations revealed severe aortic stenosis (**above**).

244 i. Pentastomids. Although worm-like in form, these parasitic organisms are actually arthropods, closely related to arachnids.
ii. Ivermectin (200mcg/kg i/m or orally, repeated after two weeks).

245 i. Gastric dilatation.
ii. Pass a stomach tube through the oesophagus to permit deflation of the gas trapped within the stomach, and instill a gas-lysing agent such as simethicone.
iii. Feeding of readily fermentable carbohydrates.

246 This vine snake had one of several soft, subcuticular lesions lanced, and a worm-like organism was found occupying each cystic space.
i. What is this organism?
ii. Is it a helminth?

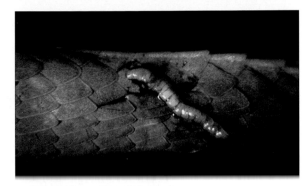

247 i. How would you interpret the whole-body radiograph of this large desert tortoise?
ii. How would you treat this condition?
iii. What is the prognosis?

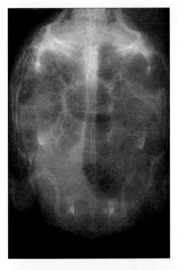

248 This is the skin and part of the shell of a box turtle.
i. What is the pale cream-coloured mass?
ii. What is its significance?
iii. How would you prevent this condition from occurring?

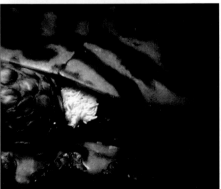

246 i. *Porocephalus* sp., a pentastomid.
ii. It is an arthropod, not a helminth.

247 i. The radiograph illustrates diffusely patchy pneumonic lung fields.
ii. A transtracheal or choanal slit specimen should be obtained for microbiological analysis and cytology, after which the tortoise should be given an appropriate bacteriocidal antibiotic, supportive fluid-replacement therapy and aggressive nursing care.
iii. Guarded. Lacking a functional diaphragm, reptiles cannot cough. Therefore, mucus-laden exudate tends to remain within the lung, becoming walled off by connective tissue and forming chronic pyogranulomata.

The figure **below** is a low-power photomicrograph of a section of lung from such an animal. Note the multiple granulomata with necrotic pus-filled centres and mixed leukocytes that have infiltrated the pulmonary parenchyma (H & E stain, x8.7 original magnification).

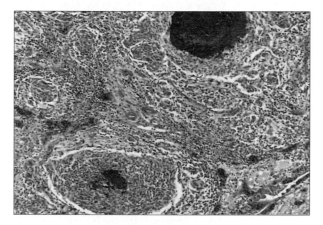

248 i. Myiasis; the mass is composed of freshly deposited flesh fly eggs.
ii. If permitted to hatch, the turtle would soon be attacked by flesh-eating maggots.
iii. Screen all cages so that flies cannot have access to the inhabitants. Also, it is good husbandry practice to inspect all captive reptiles regularly so that any problems can be detected and resolved early.

249 i. If you were examining the left eye of this rat snake what would be your diagnosis?
ii. What is the likely cause of this condition?

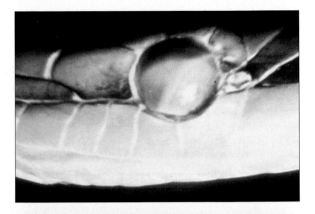

250 Reptiles are uricotelic in the manner in which their nitrogenous urinary wastes are excreted. What factors could have induced the accumulation of urate salts and, thus, hepatic, peri- and epicardial gouty deposits in this herbivorous lizard?

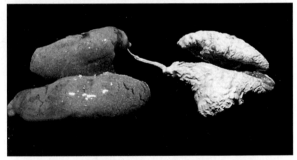

251 This radiograph shows the coelomic cavity of a mature female tegu lizard that died suddenly without displaying prior illness. What does the radiograph reveal?

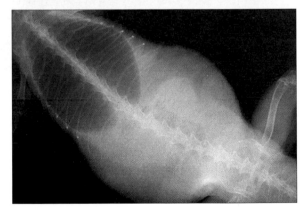

249 i. Corneal lipidosis.
ii. Cholesterol deposition secondary to trauma or hypercholesterolaemia.

250 Hyperuricaemia induced as a result of dehydration; a diet too rich in animal protein; iatrogenic aminoglycoside-induced nephrosis and visceral gout; and/or massive diffuse kidney disease leading to renal insufficiency.

251 A distended coelomic cavity and a fluid-density radiopaque mass in the right mid-coelomic region. On necropsy, a haemorrhagic right ovary was found (**below**). A branch of the right ovarian artery had ruptured spontaneously and the tegu exanguinated into the right periovarian tissues.

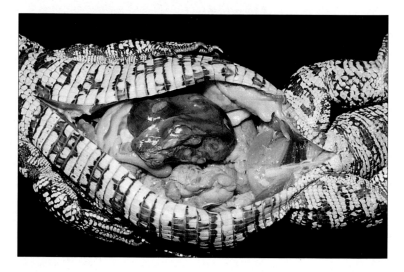

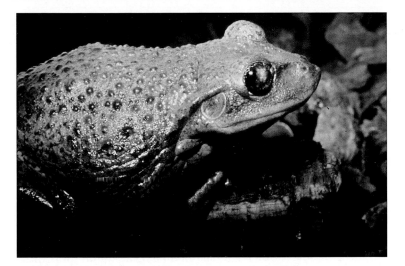

252 i. What is your diagnosis of the ocular lesion in this frog?
ii. What is the likely aetiology of this condition?
iii. How would you manage this ocular disorder?

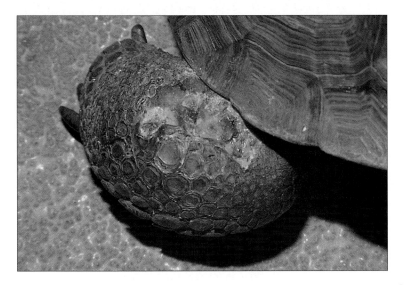

253 A Texas tortoise is shown as it appeared when presented for treatment.
i. What is your tentative diagnosis?
ii. How could the diagnosis be confirmed?

252 i. Calcium salt and cholesterol-laden deposits within the stromal layers of the cornea.

ii. Although trauma can induce this lesion, it is one which is commonly observed in captive anuran amphibians and is believed to be of dietary aetiology.

iii. As long as the frog is able to find its food prey, elective treatment is probably not necessary. If the frog's vision were to deteriorate, a partial circumferential keratectomy could be performed, followed by topical application of antibiotic medication until the cornea heals.

253 i. Massive abscessation of the right forelimb.

ii. Radiograph the affected limb; fine-needle aspiration of the swelling; cytology and/or histopathology; microbiological culture and antibiotic sensitivity testing. Note the extensive osteolysis of the humerus, radius and ulna on the radiograph (**below, left**). Chronic pyogranulomatous osteomyelitis was revealed. Microbiology yielded *Klebsiella* sp., *Aeromonas hydrophila* and *Pseudomonas aeruginosa*.

iii. The entire forelimb was amputated by scapulohumeral disarticulation. The infection was very extensive and had become well isolated by the dense fibrocollagenous connective tissue capsule (**below, right** and **bottom**). The tortoise was treated with enrofloxacin (10mg/kg daily orally for three weeks); it made an uneventful recovery learning readily to walk on its three remaining limbs.

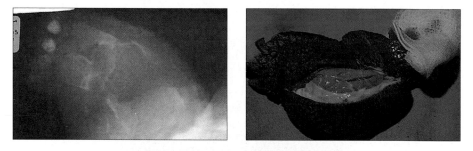

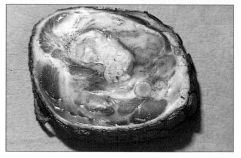

254 i. What is the ophthalmic disorder displayed by this indigo snake?
ii. How would you treat this condition?

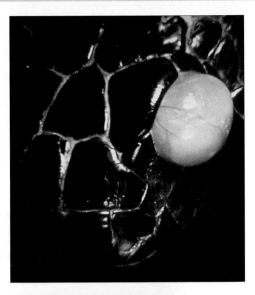

255 i. What does the dorsoventral projection, whole-body radiograph of this rhinoceros iguana reveal?
ii. What test or procedure would you perform next?
iii. How would you treat this case?
iv. How does this finding reflect on the lizard's earlier life and diet?

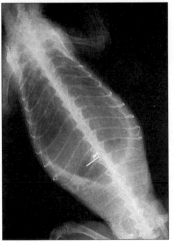

254 i. Panophthalmitis.

ii. The globe has been destroyed by the inflammatory process. Therefore, the correct treatment is to enucleate the eye and close the orbital defect with mobilised skin or, if necessary, with an antiseptic liquid plastic bandage.

255 i. Three densely radiopaque foreign objects and a metallic fastener.

ii. Take a lateral projection radiograph. Although the dorsoventral radiograph would lead one to believe that the foreign bodies are within the gastrointestinal tract, the lateral radiograph clearly reveals that the three lead-density pellets are embedded alongside and beneath the spine, and that the nail-like fastener is located well above the stomach and adjacent to the last ribs, just barely penetrating into the soft tissues of the epaxial muscle mass.

iii. Surgical exploration, making certain that a wide area of the lizard's dorsal, lateral and ventral integumentary surfaces are prepared for surgery. Three shotgun pellets and a copper nail were found and removed from the epaxial and subvertebral muscles; the nail was encased in a fibrous connective tissue capsule and was surrounded with pus (**below**). A healed penetrating wound was found in the wall of the stomach where the nail had perforated the gastric tunics.

iv. The shotgun pellets suggest that this iguana had been hatched and had grown to at least near adulthood in its wild habitat rather than having been hatched in captivity.

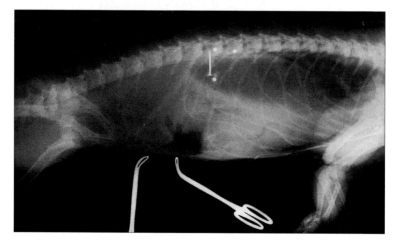

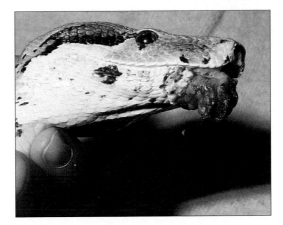

256 A mature boa constrictor was examined because an expanding mass had developed from the soft tissues lining its mandible. This mass caused substantial deformity.
i. What is your diagnosis?
ii. How would you confirm the diagnosis?
iii. How would you treat this condition?
iv. What is the prognosis?

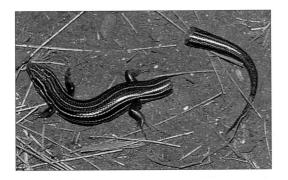

257 You are presented with an insectivorous skink for routine examination. You reach into the terrarium in which the skink is housed and carefully lift it out. As you are holding the skink gently and just about to transfer the beloved pet to the examination table, its tail suddenly breaks off and it falls to the floor of the cage and wriggles continuously for the next 10 minutes as its horrified owner gazes back and forth from the now-shed tail to you, becoming ever more doleful and dispirited.
i. Now that your self-confidence and 'bedside manner' have been utterly shattered, what should you do?
ii. What should you tell the now-angry owner of the skink with the unexpectedly truncated tail?

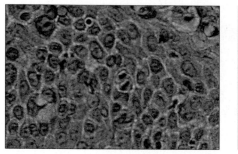 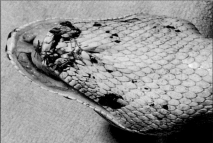

256 i. Well-differentiated squamous cell carcinoma.
ii. Fine-needle or wedge biopsy and histological examination of stained tissue sections (**above, left**). Note the intercellular bridges that characterise keratinocytes and help establish that this tumour is of squamous cell origin.
iii. Total excision, including a cuff of normal-appearing integument surrounding the mass (**above, right**). Radiotherapy should be considered in selected cases.
iv. Fair to good, depending upon the aggressive behaviour of the tumour. In this instance, the boa is still alive and thriving more than six years following excision.

257 i. Once the tail has autotomised fully, there is no treatment that will restore its viability because the blood supply to the appendage is irreparably disrupted. The blood vessels serving the tail go into immediate spasm which prevents substantial blood loss or traumatic shock.
ii. Many lizards (and a very few snakes) have 'break points' in their caudal vertebrae which permit the tail to be voluntarily shed when the lizard (or snake) perceives that it is in danger of predation or capture. Even very mild manual restraint (or even the threat of restraint) often results in a lizard autotomising its tail. The tail usually begins to regenerate within a few months and, after a year or two, the regrown tail is almost as long and thick as the original – although its scale pattern and colour may not quite match the former appearance. (Spontaneous caudal autotomy usually elicits equal consternation by both the pet's owner and the handler who was responsible for the tail loss. To the former, a previously perfect pet or specimen has now acquired a major blemish; to the latter, the occurrence has been a shocking demonstration of the vagaries of exotic animal practice!)

Index